DENTAL HYGIENE:

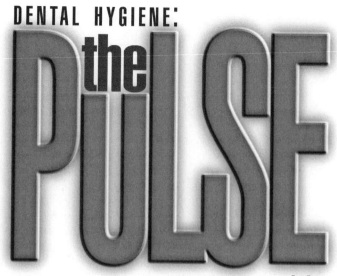

the PULSE

of the
PRACTICE

DENTAL HYGIENE:

the PULSE

of the PRACTICE

Cynthia McKane - Wagester

Dental Economics

RDH
THE NATIONAL MAGAZINE FOR DENTAL HYGIENE PROFESSIONALS

PennWell

Copyright © 2002 by
PennWell Corporation
1421 S. Sheridan Road
Tulsa, Oklahoma 74112
800-752-9764
sales@pennwell.com
www.pennwell-store.com
www.pennwell.com

cover design by Clark Bell
book design by Amy Spehar

Library of Congress Cataloging-in-Publication Data Pending
McKane-Wagester, Cynthia.
    Dental hygiene : the pulse of the practice / Cynthia (Cindy) McKane-Wagester.
        p. ; cm. -- (Dental economics)
    ISBN 0-87814-711-X
        1. Dental hygiene. 2. Dental hygienists. 3. Interprofessional relations. 4. Dentistry.
    I. Title: Pulse of the practice. II. Title. III. Dental economics (Tulsa, Okla.)
        [DNLM: 1. Oral Hygiene. 2. Dental Hygienists. 3. Dentists. 4. Interprofessional
    Relations. 5. Practice Management, Dental. WU 113 M478d 2002]
    RK60.7 .M38 2002
    607.6'01--dc21

                                                                            2002022088

Printed in the United States of America

1   2   3   4   5   06   05   04   03   02

Contents

Acknowledgements

Dental Hygiene: The Pulse of the Practice could not have been written without the encouragement and support of Dr. Woody Oakes, who has been a mentor and a friend through good times and bad.

Inspiration for the direction of this work came from Walter Hailey and Steve Anderson, whose philosophy on life and dentistry so closely matches my own.

A special word of thanks goes to my friend and colleague, Mark Hartley, who graciously agreed to write the preface to this book before seeing the first draft, and to Dr. Ian Shuman, who nudges me to move forward and challenges me to see things in a different light.

Special thanks is also due to Anne Marie Evans, who held down the fort at McKane & Associates while I sat at the computer, and to Tamara Cornelison, who made sure that every pronoun matched its antecedent.

To Kirk Bjornsgaard belongs the credit for allaying my anxiety that things would never be done in time.

Above all, I thank my husband Ken and my daughter Ashley, whose love and understanding make everything possible.

Preface

You're obviously focused on this page for the moment, but I'd like to talk about a couple of forces that don't seem to be on the same page, figuratively speaking—the restorative operatory and the hygiene operatory.

Dental schools today are more aware of the fact that this woman shows up in their graduates' offices and says, "Hi, I'm the hygienist. Whassup?"

If you ever want to see the expression of a clueless person, check out the face of a new dentist who has his or her first encounter with a dental hygienist.

As hinted above, though, many dental schools are incorporating a local dental hygiene program into the education process, forcing students from both schools to get acquainted at the earliest stages. This professional partnership launches many dental practices into a calm sea where every aspect of treatment clicks together beautifully. A dynamic duo of a dentist and a hygienist is an extremely productive relationship that accomplishes everything from teaching a young child to use a toothbrush to saving the life of an adult patient who has an undiagnosed cancerous lesion. Together, they bring a special meaning to healthcare team.

However, this type of partnership doesn't happen often enough; there's often a "rocky start" involved. Dentists and hygienists often engage in a learning curve that's frequently painful to watch. It's such a shame too, since each has so much to offer to the other, as well as the clients and the communities they serve.

It shouldn't be this way, and Cynthia McKane-Wagester knows this. Cindy has put together an excellent primer on the integration of restorative and preventive dentistry. Within these pages, everyone gets on the same page about the role of the doctor and hygienist in the contemporary dental practice.

Mark Hartley
Editor,
RDH magazine

Introduction

THE EVOLUTION OF DENTAL HYGIENE

Dental hygiene is the field of dentistry that is based on preserving and maintaining oral health. Concerned with keeping the teeth and gums in healthy condition, dental hygiene is more and more defined in terms of preventive care that provides protection against oral diseases as well as other diseases that affect the human body.

The history of dental hygiene is a long and winding road that is inextricably intertwined with the history of dentistry and the history of medicine from the earliest days of human concern with pain and health and healing. Through archeological findings, records of ancient civilizations provide some interesting, albeit incomplete, information about dental health concerns. As early as 5000 B.C., Sumerian physicians, attempting to ascertain the cause of tooth decay that plagued their patients, theorized that it was caused by a "tooth worm." Their theory was accepted well into the first century by the ancient Romans, who treated toothaches with the smoke of burning henbane plants. It was believed that the smoke would suffocate tooth worms and end the problem.

Ancient Egyptians prided themselves on specializing in various fields of medicine. Some specialized in tooth and gum diseases; in fact, records dating back to 3000 B.C. refer to a "Chief Toother" in one of the royal households whose functions included ameliorating the pain associated with decaying teeth. Ancient Chinese physicians were treating pain caused by tooth decay with acupuncture as early as 2500 B.C. Perhaps most intriguing are records from ancient Assyrian physicians who seem to have understood to some degree that diseased teeth were related to systemic ailments, a theory closely related to modern perceptions of oral health.

Centuries later, Hippocrates, the Greek physician who is considered the father of medicine in Western civilization, also wrote about diseases of the teeth. But both he and Galen, another noted Greek physician, believed that decay came from internal inflammation caused by the ubiquitous tooth worm first "discovered" by the ancient Sumerians.

In the eighth century, the world of medicine was revolutionized by Arabian physicians, some of whom developed an interest in dental therapeutics. Avicenna, the personal physician to the Sultan of Bukhara, warned about damage to tooth enamel caused by caustic dentrifices. He wrote about this and other medical theories in what can be viewed as the first version of a medical encyclopedia, which was used throughout the Middle East, and then in Western Europe, as a reliable source of medical information well into the fifteenth century.

Another Arab physician, Abulcasis of Cordoba, was a great surgeon. His writings became the basis for surgical education in early European medical schools. Advocating a holistic approach to keeping the body healthy, Abulcasis devoted a portion of his voluminous writing to the care and treatment of teeth as a means of promoting total health.

In the medieval west, eastern ideas on dental therapeutics flourished and then faded away as religious intolerance and social instability encouraged superstition and moved systematic scientific research into a shady background. Despite information readily available in the writings of eastern physicians and theorists, Western European physicians and surgeons of the sixteenth century began promoting the idea that tooth decay was caused by "bad blood." The recommended treatment was a combination of voodoo-type incantations and bloodletting. Preventing tooth decay was not considered—the thrust was entirely on getting rid of a painful problem.

In seventeenth century colonial America, preventive dentistry was also nearly unheard of. People developed toothaches and teeth were pulled, not by doctors, but by barbers or blacksmiths. This approach to dentistry—focused on problem-solving rather than problem prevention—stayed securely in place until the nineteenth century, when physicians and others who were interested in toothaches and other oral disorders began to understand that decay was caused from the outside, not by mysterious internal inflammation, tooth worms, or bad blood. They "discovered," in essence, that eating, while necessary to sustain life, made people susceptible to tooth decay.

A pioneer in this area was a New Orleans dentist named Levi Parmly, who made the connection between food particles left on and between teeth with the accumulation of tartar on tooth surfaces, which eventually led to red and sore gums. He encouraged a preventive approach as an antidote— regular cleansing of the teeth and gums. Among the preventive measures he advocated were brushing with salt and cleaning between teeth with a waxed silk thread, the precursor of today's dental floss.

Modern American dentistry as we know it today got its start almost by accident with two dentists who believed that the entire body was affected by oral health. When Dr. Horace H. Hayden and Dr. Harris Aaron Chapin proposed to lecture on their theories at the University of Maryland, they were ignored or denounced by their medical contemporaries. Because they expounded ideas considered radical by some and inconsequential by others, their request to present their theories in the formal university setting was summarily dismissed as ambitious over-reaching.

Undaunted, Hayden and Chapin refused to bow to the collective wisdom and traditionalist stagnation of their stuffy medical cousins. In 1840, they established the Baltimore College of Dental Surgery. The college, the first of its kind in the world, was granted a charter by the Maryland General Assembly. It provided the dental profession with something it had never had—a formal institution of learning, devoted solely to the education and training of students intending to practice dentistry.

With the establishment of the Baltimore College of Dental Surgery, dentistry was given an official stamp of approval as one of the respectable professions. In time, the theories of preventive oral care—dental hygiene— were also recognized, digested, and accepted. One of the earliest printed records of this acceptance can be found in the transcript of the proceedings of the American Dental Association (ADA) meeting held in 1870. One of the resolutions passed at the meeting was to encourage publishers of schoolbooks for American children to disseminate information on dental hygiene to those children by including in their school texts helpful and informative materials about proper oral health care.

In the following decades, preventive oral health care became increasingly popular, and dentists throughout the country began to focus increasing attention to prophylaxis as an essential aspect of their practices.

Dental hygiene now had its place in the profession, but until 1913, it was the responsibility and function of the dentist. All this changed when a Connecticut dentist named Alfred C. Fones developed an interest in prophylaxis for children. His interest developed into a passion, and his passion developed into a distinct specialty in the field of dentistry. While devoting himself to preventive oral care for children, Fones trained his assistant in prophylaxis. That assistant, Irene Newman, became the prototype for today's professional registered dental hygienist (RDH). She was the first of a small group of dental hygienists trained by Fones to perform some of the most basic prophylactic procedures that hygienists perform to this day.

Other trainees learned the procedures at the Fones Clinic for Dental Hygienists that was officially opened in 1913. His first classes were taught in his garage; his first faculty, all handpicked, top-notch dentists and reputable professors of dentistry, were volunteers. They worked without pay to promote an idea they shared with Fones: the need for a professional dental healthcare giver specifically trained in preventive oral health care.

Connecticut passed a law licensing hygienists in 1917. Other states soon followed suit. In 1923, the American Dental Hygiene Association (ADHA) was founded and dental hygienists were given a professional organization to call their own, one that provided resources, information, and group identity to the growing number of fledgling hygienists throughout the country.

For these early dental hygienists, all women, career opportunities were severely limited by tradition, custom, and gender bias. They began practicing as preventive oral health professionals mostly with schoolchildren. When the resulting improvements in the dental health of children treated by these hygienists became apparent, some in the dental community began to notice and accept their work as a valuable contribution to the field. But acceptance was slow, and the scope of the hygienist's influence in the dental community was constrained by resistance to change.

Education on prevention was in its infancy and, as an evolving science, it was accepted by some and suspected by many. Limited and sometimes primitive instrumentation presented its own set of problems. Some dentists, wary of sharing their professional limelight with anyone, were reluctant to introduce hygienists into their practices. Some did so grudgingly and condescendingly. Early hygienists worked for low pay and low esteem; as women in a field dominated by male dentists, their responsibilities were not always related to hygiene. Many were expected to perform clerical functions and housekeeping functions as well. These conditions persisted even after states instituted formal licensing and ADHA activists established national standards for the profession.

The Dental Hygienist Today

Today's dental hygienist, the descendant of the 27 graduates of Alfred Fones' first class, is a bird of different plumage, a bird that has spread its wings and soared to heights and distances that her predecessors could not have imagined. She is better educated and better equipped. She is almost universally respected for her professional skills and is increasingly more involved in the diagnosis and treatment of oral health conditions. As a graduate of a school of dental hygiene that has been accredited by the ADA, she has studied microbiology, chemistry, pathology, anatomy, and physiology. She has passed state and national examinations that have qualified her for certification and licensing. The range of her clinical skills has increased enormously, and the range of her other responsibilities has increased proportionately.

On any given day, today's hygienist will perform a soft tissue exam, apply fluoride and other caries-preventive agents, provide dietary counseling, and appear as a guest speaker at a community dental health program. She will perform scaling and root planing and will routinely screen patients for oral cancer. She is expected to be proficient in the operation of dental x-ray equipment, and to expertly expose, process, and interpret radiographic images. She is expected to monitor patient health history with the same practiced and efficient capability as she monitors inventory in her operatory. She is, as well, expected to understand the value of knowledge, and her commitment to continuing education is as great as her commitment to the well being of her patients. In some states, she may be expected to administer local anesthetics and general analgesia, place and carve filling materials, and perform many additional periodontal procedures.

Career opportunities and venues for dental hygienists are abundant. Once limited to classroom settings or private practices where she was often viewed as a general assistant who could be counted on to chip in with the broom after chipping away at the tartar, she can now choose to work almost anywhere. Today's dental hygienists can be found in a private practice, a clinic, a hospital, private industry, a correctional facility, a Health Maintenance Organization (HMO), and even aboard a cruise ship.

Whatever the location, today's hygienist is one of the most valuable members of a dental team, and the dental hygiene department, whether it consists of one hygienist or twelve, is the single most important component of any dental practice. It is in the hygiene chair where most patients will be introduced to a practice and in the hygiene chair where patients will form their most lasting impression of that practice. It is in the hygiene operatory where the most prevalent oral health problem in America—periodontal disease—is diagnosed, prevented, or treated. It is in the hygiene operatory where other oral health or overall health concerns are discovered and monitored and re-directed, if need be, to other departments or other dental or medical healthcare professionals.

Unfortunately, there is more than a little truth in the time-honored adage that the more things change, the more things stay the same.

Today there are more than 200 dental hygiene schools in the United States and more than 100,000 hygienists. In some practices, the role of the hygienist is becoming increasingly more important—from the perspective of health and from the perspective of business. In too many others, however, the role of the hygienist has remained focused on the simplest and most primitive aspect of dental hygiene—chipping away at plaque and tartar and dispensing free samples of toothpaste to adults and smiley-face stickers to children.

In a country that has prided itself on providing its citizens with the best health care in the entire world, this last is shamefully inadequate. It is especially problematic in light of the recent report of the United States Surgeon

General, which has confirmed once and for all that the mouth is indeed connected to the body and that the state of oral health in this country verges on deplorable.

Thus, it is the definition, or re-definition, of the dental hygienist that is the focus of this book. It is a re-definition that, by extension, hopes to redefine the profession of dentistry as a whole by providing a step-by-step analysis of practice restructuring that is attuned to the concept of the dental hygiene department as the *Pulse of the Practice*—an untapped and still under-valued resource that can be enhanced and developed for the mutual benefit of dental practitioners and dental patients alike.

1 In the Beginning . . .

> *The beginning is the most*
> *important part of the work. — Plato*

For many years, too many in the dental profession viewed the dental hygienist as a necessary evil. On the one hand, dentists knew that they needed a dental hygienist. On the other hand, they saw the hygienist and her department as the money pit of their practices, one that swallowed hundreds and thousands of dollars each year in salaries, supplies, high tech equipment, and assorted other expenses that made the department's profitability quotient redder than anyone liked.

For numerous reasons, more and more dental practitioners are beginning to question the validity of the old image of the dental hygiene department. The profession is slowly beginning to view dental hygiene as a long undervalued investment that, with a little patience and some smart work, can pay off handsomely.

While the dental care profession is at long last giving the dental hygiene department the second look it deserves, most individual practices have not yet learned how to tap into its true potential. In truth, very few practices have developed a master strategy for revamping the department to meet the needs of today's business environment. Most dental practices have a far too general approach. Their strategies for reassessment, reorientation, and readjustment are unfocused and haphazard. They try this idea or that idea and become frustrated when the hygiene department page of the account ledger continues to bleed. Some give up. Some continue a hit or miss approach, hoping to find the secret formula. Some take the patchwork approach, assuming that if they fix this or renovate that, everything else will magically fall into place. All too few recognize that the secret begins with scrapping all the old misconceptions and creating an entirely new design.

This new design begins with seeing the dental hyiene department as it relates to the business of dentistry. Above all, this means recognizing that dentistry is a business. There are bills and salaries to be paid, and unless you are practicing as a dental missionary in the wilds of Borneo, part of the reason you practice dentistry is to make money. For too many people, this simple truth is difficult to admit, let alone discuss. But making a decision to transform your hygiene department into a department that is more productive means having the integrity to understand that the underlying motive is profitability. Having looked the truth in the face, we can now examine it in detail.

PROFIT AND PRODUCTIVITY

In most practices, the hygiene department (or the hygienist) is limited by custom, habit, tradition, or shortsightedness to providing nothing more than routine maintenance. But a hygiene department that offers nothing more than tooth cleaning is neither productive nor profitable. For a hygiene department to be truly the pulse of the practice, it has to produce and generate dentistry far beyond the traditional scope. If your program is well planned and well executed, it can increase the hygiene department's production as much as 50% per month, increase the number of hygiene appointments beyond your most optimistic estimates, and improve acceptance percentages for the entire practice. A single hygienist, with the proper motivation and the proper environment, can produce approximately between $800 and $1,200 or more each day. Creating the motivation and the environment comes first.

All good dental healthcare providers recognize that their most important goal is to provide excellent care for their patients. As professionals in the business of dentistry, they also recognize that their practices thrive in direct proportion to the number of patients who come (and come back) to their offices. The relationship between productivity and profit is obvious: giving your patients the best means everyone wins. You make this happen by setting goals. You achieve the goals when you have the vision to make them work. Combining your vision and your goals into a mission statement provides a path to follow. It defines the purpose and philosophy of your practice.

Applying these concepts to an entire practice is important. Applying them to the dental hygiene department is a tactical maneuver that can make profitability soar. Consider, for example, the benefits of a hygiene department with its own goals, its own vision, and its own mission statement. Productivity goals can be identified and set by the people who are in the best position to define those goals, set realistic deadlines for those goals, and monitor the success rate for those goals. Identifying goals and objectives provides them with a sense of direction and keeps them focused. Making decisions on how to achieve those goals by implementing workable strategies empowers vision. A departmental mission statement will reflect the goals, the vision, and the departmental philosophy.

There may be, initially, some concern about granting the members of the hygiene department too much autonomy. Will this result in chaos? Will the goals and the vision and the philosophy contradict the goals and vision and philosophy of the practice? Will I lose control? All of these questions can be answered with a resounding "no." When given the opportunity, most people will live up to what you expect of them. If you expect the best, you will get the best.

The members of your dental hygiene team know they are employees in your dental practice. If you have hired them and trained them and given them an understanding of your own practice goals, visions, and philosophy, they are unlikely to let you down by creating something so divergent that it will make the practice collapse. In fact, their ideas may make you review, modify, and update your own. Vesting in them the authority to be responsible for the success of the department gives them a sense of autonomy and instills in them a professional pride. Invariably, this results in initiative and enthusiasm that are proactive and positive. It creates the proverbial win-win situation for all concerned.

VISION

Vision is the art of
seeing things invisible.
— JONATHAN SWIFT

In the Broadway musical *Kismet,* the hero is a nobody who aspires to greatness. Wooing the sultan's favor while he woos the sultan's daughter, he philosophizes in song about the difference between those who succeed and those who settle. His metaphorical analysis begins with overhearing a fool spouting words of wisdom while sitting under an olive tree:

Munching on an olive, the fool proclaims that life would be so much better if he had an entire olive tree. He then considers how much better everything would be if he could have an entire grove of olive trees. The flight of fancy carries him to an even more exciting conclusion -- contemplating the enormous range of possibilities open to him if he could have the entire world.

The fool, exhausted by the depth of his own words, falls asleep. The hero, taking the words to heart, experiences "a wondrous change" and begins to see the world as a place where all things are possible. He discovers the power of vision.

Vision *does* make all things possible. Without vision, the passion to succeed cannot sustain itself, because it has no shape and no direction. Having vision, on the other hand, means knowing what kind of dentistry you want to offer, knowing what is best for your patients, and knowing how the hygiene department fits into the great scheme of things. It means having the integrity to see what needs to be changed, improved, resolved, restructured, or abandoned.

If you envision a master practice with a master dental hygiene department at its heart, the images of where you want to be should be even clearer and more specific. You must first define (or redefine) your vision of a successful master practice. You must define dentistry as a commitment to a philosophy of excellence. You must define how you perceive the business of dentistry. And then you must define the role of the hygiene department as it relates to all of these. It is only when you have clearly and specifically visualized all of these components that you can set realistic goals that reflect your mission and your purpose and your practice philosophy.

SETTING GOALS

When you embark on something,
fix your intentions and selfishness
behind you, then you cannot fail
— MIYAMOTO MUSASHI.
THE BOOK OF FIVE RINGS (1596)

Goal setting gives you a sense of direction and keeps you focused. It also prevents you from feeling frustrated. For you to have any chance of achieving your goals, they must be written down. If you don't commit your goals to paper, they are not goals.

Each of us has social and family goals as well as business and financial goals. If you are serious about making the dental hygiene department the pulse of your master practice, you must create goals that will make the department function in a manner that will complement your vision.

Your primary goal, then, should be to restructure your dental hygiene department so that it promotes the business of dentistry while adhering to a commitment to the philosophy of excellence. Setting specific goals within this general goal is the next step. Focus on hiring and training productive and effective dental team members to improve quality, consistency, and optimal dentistry. Focus on improving scheduling for optimal productivity. Focus on monitoring hygiene statistics so that you can improve practice statistics. Focus on improving treatment procedures, patient education, and marketing strategies. Make sure that your goals include a commitment to minimizing broken appointments and cancellations. Make sure that your goals include establishing a healthy reactivation program and a successful periodontal program.

As every one of these objectives suggests, what happens or doesn't happen in the hygiene department has an impact on the entire dental practice. The hygiene department, for better or worse, affects patient flow, atmosphere, customer service, and marketing. All of these factors translate to practice productivity and profitability. Measure the pulse of the hygiene department and you measure the health of the practice. A practice with a strong hygiene department will flourish. A practice with a weak hygiene department will flounder. It's as simple as that.

ACHIEVING GOALS

Fortune sides with him who dares.
—VIRGIL

Before any attempt at implementation, make certain that the goals you have set for your practice and the goals of your hygiene department are compatible. If there is any question about this, something needs to be reviewed and revised for consistency. If the goals are harmonious, they will be easier to achieve and will enhance each other. If the goals clash, no amount of work will produce the desired results.

Having identified and refined your goals, define your strategies for accomplishing each of them. Set a time or date for when goals should be accomplished, giving each one no more than a year. Identify the person who is responsible for each strategy related to achieving each goal, remembering always that you are the person in charge and that the ultimate responsibility is yours.

Keep your goals realistic and keep them fresh and alive by reminding yourself, in detail, how you will benefit once they have been achieved. Make a point of writing down, as vividly as you can, what will happen if you don't meet your goals. Try to describe the changes in your life that will happen in one year, five years, and ten years, both if you do achieve your goals and if you don't. How will this affect you, your business, and your family? By creating a realistic understanding of the pain you will have if you fail, and conversely, the pleasure you will have if you succeed, your motivation will increase exponentially.

Evaluate your results and then evaluate your methods. If your original strategy did not work, learn from it and be prepared to embrace change. Successful people recognize that something is not working and recognize that the flaw is often in the methodology and seldom in the goal. They are not afraid to experiment with new and different and sometimes untried approaches, and this is often the difference between failure and success. Go boldly and confidently, but never forget the difference between a calculated risk and a blind leap of faith prompted by panic.

Realize that growth comes from all types of experiences and be positive. Understand that problems will arise, and remind yourself that problems are meant to be solved. Assigning blame is worthless and counterproductive. Instead, challenge yourself to find workable solutions.

Above all, choose wisely your response to a goal achieved. Celebrate it and celebrate the vision that made it happen. Relish it. Enjoy it. Commend yourself and all those responsible for a job well done. Then raise your standards and their standards by setting a new goal.

DEVELOPING A PURPOSE

Whether you are a seasoned professional or a novice just ready to begin your journey, you must constantly nurture your commitment to your profession. Keeping your passion fresh and vital is essential. With passion, you will remain enthusiastic and focused about what you are doing. You will truly be able to identify your purpose and articulate that purpose within a philosophy that has meaning.

Remember that the most important purpose you have is a commitment to excellence. Excellence means striving to be the best that you can be, even if you don't perform perfectly. If you strive to do things to the best of your ability, surround yourself with good people, and treat your patients with care and consideration, then you cannot fail. More than anything else, you must *desire* to be the best. By maintaining a clear vision of the difference dentistry can make in someone's lifestyle and health, you'll take advantage of every opportunity to give patients what they truly need. When you are true to your commitment to excellence, you will have happier and healthier patients and your purpose will have been served.

Having vision makes a goal attainable. You achieve the goal when you have the vision to make it work. Now bring goals and purpose and vision together and you have a philosophy. This philosophy defines you and your work. It should be written down as a mission statement.

Developing a Philosophy of Practice and the Importance of a Written Mission Statement

Just as it is true that no two people are exactly alike, it is also true that no two people have exactly the same basic philosophy. It is extremely important, however, to know what your philosophy is and to ascertain that the philosophy of your hygiene department is on the same wavelength. Take the time to think this issue through, because a clearly defined philosophy provides the "passion" power for your personal and professional development. Divergent philosophies within a practice can wreak terminal havoc.

For both the practice and the hygiene department, a strong sense of mission is essential if objectives are to be met. Everyone must know what is going on. Without a clear and complete picture of purpose or direction, you will simply tread water instead of progressing and growing. Then ask yourself how your purpose reflects your vision and your objectives. Are the purpose and direction of the hygiene department on the same track? Your answer should be a resounding yes, because goals, purpose, and direction are a mirror of your philosophy of practice. Write it down and you have created a mission statement.

Some statements of mission are very short: "It is my purpose to assist every patient to achieve a lifetime of dental health." Some are more inclusive: "My purpose is to help achieve a state of optimal dental and oral health personally appropriate for each patient. By continually striving to provide excellence in personal and professional service in a caring and gentle manner, I enhance the quality of my patients' lives."

A person who has a written mission statement reflecting a sense of purpose and a philosophy of practice is in a very strong position. When you know who you are, it is much easier to know what to do in each and every situation. The same holds true for the practice and the departments within the practice, especially the hygiene department that is its heart and soul.

A truly effective mission statement should include a declaration about quality, excellence, and efficiency. It should also reflect your position regarding honesty, integrity, and fairness in dealing with clients. Dentistry has a code of ethics; everyone *must* be held accountable to it.

A good mission statement should define the kind of atmosphere you want to create within your practice. Remember that the dental team plays the most important role in the success of your practice. Remember that no one ever becomes successful by doing only what is required. Raise your standards and give more of yourself. Expect the members of your team to do the same. Then all of you will achieve the success you deserve.

2 Transitions

Change is good, but the process of turning the "hygiene department" into the "pulse of the practice" will come with its share of growing pains. Getting from vision to substance is never easy. If you begin with vision, you will find the right road, but it will truly be the road less traveled. You will find yourself breaking with tradition, defying conventional wisdom, and contradicting the self-anointed experts who say it can't be done. You will often find yourself defending your vision to colleagues who firmly believe that the road you are taking is nothing but a dead-end street. The only way to prove them wrong is to have the courage to believe in your vision and proceed with the certainty that the road you have chosen is the right road for you and your practice.

One of the most important lessons you and members of your hygiene department will be learning at this time is to recognize your own value. Details in the dental healthcare profession translate to numbers, statistics, percentages, ratios, and dollar amounts. There are specific vital signs that should be monitored in a well-run and profitable dental hygiene department. They include gross production, production per hour, collection percentage, receivables ratio, new patient appointments, average new patient treatment potential, case acceptance ratio, treatment completion rate, and recall or recare rate.

For this reason, the first step of the journey is to take a good look at where you are. Simply stated, you must know the current score of your practice and your hygiene department before you can make changes and improvements. Evaluate the total practice first. (Figs. 2-1, 2-2, and 2-3)

Vital signs for a healthy practice:
Vital sign/healthy range for the dentist

- Dentist's production per hour - $300 +
- Accounts receivable – one-half of one month's production
- True receivables – 0–90 days
  0–60 – 75%
  61–90 – 25%
- Consistent flow of new patients – Average 10–20 per month
- Retention of 90% of patients annually
- Recare effectiveness of 85% or better
- Less than 10% loss through broken appointments monthly
- Collections 96-98% of production annually
- 80% scheduling effectiveness monthly
- 800 to 1,000 patient base (active, non-managed care)
- 80% case acceptance of dentistry presented
- Power block scheduling (two–four each day)
- Three internal marketing plans and three external marketing plans in place at any given time

Vital signs for a healthy practice:
Vital sign/healthy range for the dental hygienist

- Hygienists' production per hour is $125+
- 100% of patients should pre-appoint for their continuing care appointments (check with special insurance)

- Up to 75% of patients can or could be referred to a more frequent recare return
- Up to 50% of patients can be referred to some level of a periodontal program
- Less than 10% loss through cancellations or broken appointments monthly
- 40-80% of doctor treatment coming out of the hygiene recare chairs monthly
- Retention of 90% of patients annually through the hygiene department
- Power block booking – two–three a day

Vision of practice defined? _____ Mission and purpose? _____ Goals set? _____
Operatories: Total _____ Doctor _____ Hygiene _____Other_____
Are they equally equipped? Yes_____ No_____
Staff size: Hygienists _____ CDAs _____ DAs _____ Office Admin. _____
Other_____
What style of practice do you have? _____
What percentage of your practice are children? _____
Do you accept any HMO/reduced fee?_____What are the percentages?
HMO _____ PPO _____
Traditional third-party _____ Fee for service _____
How many patients (seen in hygiene within the last year) do you have
in your practice? _____
When did you last complete a chart audit? _____
How many total hygiene days per week? (Count two hygienists on one day
as two days.) _____
On the average, how many patients do your hygienists see per day? _____
Are you scheduling on a 10- or 15-minute unit? _____
Are cancellations and failures an issue in the hygiene schedule? _____
To what degree? _____
Does the hygienist "co-assess" with the doctor during each recare exam? _____
How many weeks does the hygienist work per year? _____
How many new adult patients do you see per month on average? _____
Does the hygienist see new patients? _____

Figure 2–1 Practice/Hygiene Analysis Form

What are your fees for the following procedures?
- Adult prophylaxis   _____
- Root planing per quadrant   _____
- Periodontal maintenance   _____
- 4 Bitewings   _____
- 2 Bitewings   _____
- Examination (Periodic)   _____
- FMX   _____
- Child prophylaxis   _____
- Initial examination   _____
- Panorex   _____
- Fluoride treatment   _____
- Irrigation   _____
- Complete radiographic series   _____

What was the date of your last fee increase? _____

How often do you take bitewings? _____ Panorex _____ FMX _____

Do you have a radiographic policy? _____

What is the average monthly production in hygiene? _____

Does this production include examinations and x-rays that the hygienist may take?

_____

How are your hygienists paid? _____

Reviewing your procedure analysis report, how many of the following procedures have been performed year-to-date?

Veneers	_____	Crowns	_____	Onlays	_____
Adult prophylaxis	_____	Gross debridement	_____	Fluoride irrigation	_____
Root planing	_____	Adult Pro	_____	Periodontal examination	_____
4 Bitewings	_____	Periodontal (4910)	_____	Panorex	_____
Examinations	_____	2 Bitewings	_____	Whitening	_____
Child Prophylaxis	_____	FMX	_____	Antibiotic Therapy	_____

Who is in charge of the recare program? _____

Figure 2–1 continued

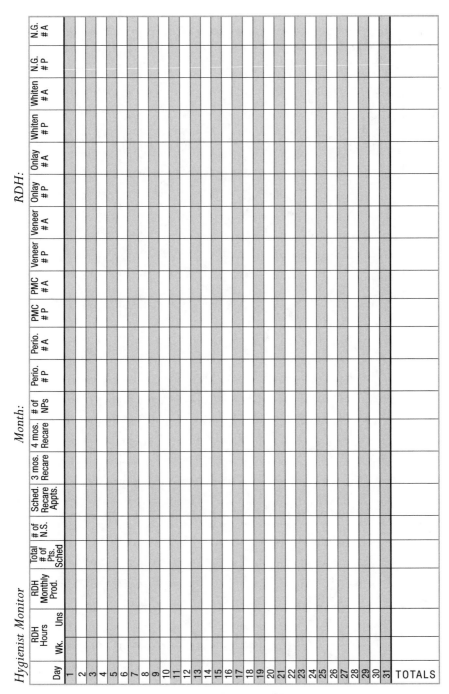

Figure 2–2 Hygienist Monitor

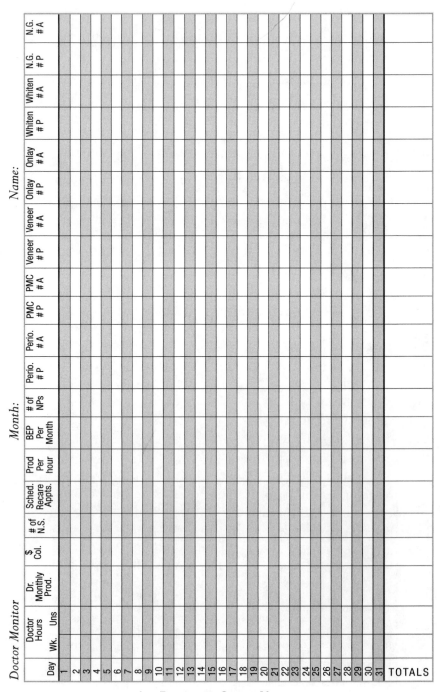

Figure 2–3 Doctor Monitor

Once you have determined where you are, you can begin to move forward, and the best way to do this is to use the information you have collected as a base from which to *visualize* where you want to be. *Visualize* the hygiene department as the pulse of the practice even though you are outnumbered and outgunned. This is the key to actualization—the one that can make all the difference between success and mediocrity. Work *with* your dental hygiene department to develop its goals and vision and philosophy. Do this by providing information and guidance. Make sure everyone in the department knows what kind of dentistry you want to offer in your practice, what is best for the patients in your practice, and how the hygiene department fits into the grand scheme of things. It is in their best interest to work with you on this and they will.

Visualize preventive maintenance visits (PMV) that are more than just cleanings. Because statistics show that that more than 75% of the nation's adults suffer from some form of periodontal disease, the PMV can be one of the valuable tools in increasing practice productivity and profitability. If one of the goals of the practice and the department is helping patients keep their teeth for a lifetime, everyone needs to see the PMV as more than a session with a tooth picker. It should be *visualized* as a session with a capable and skilled professional who can recognize all stages of periodontal disease, can recommend a periodontal treatment program, and can educate the patient in a way that makes the patient recognize that the treatment is valuable and necessary.

In light of the report issued in 2000 by the office of the United States Surgeon General, a strong and vital hygiene department is more critical than ever. Neglecting or ignoring oral health can cause grievous illnesses, worsen other illness, and even lead to death. As healthcare providers, we are committed to healing patients, not just cavities. Thus, it is neither ghoulish nor mercenary for a hygiene department to capitalize on these facts. *Visualize* a hygiene department where patients are thoroughly educated about proper oral health care, preventive and corrective, and begin to truly understand the value of the dentistry offered in your practice.

Finally, *visualize* a hygiene department that can monitor its own numbers, use those numbers to set appropriate goals, and design an agenda for meeting those goals.

When all of these components work harmoniously, the hygiene department can improve every aspect of the practice. *Visualize* improved case acceptance and lower rates of cancellations and broken appointments. *Visualize* improved customer service and patient education that leads to an 85% or better recare rate. *Visualize* at least a 50% increase in the number of patients referred to a more intensive level of periodontal treatment. Then *visualize* how everyone associated with the practice—you, your patients, your staff, and your community—will benefit. It is at this point that you will stop looking back over your shoulder and wondering about what has been left behind. Your focus will be on the horizon and on the steps you will be taking along the road that leads to success.

A Word about Motivation

There are three kinds of people
in this world:
Those who make it happen
Those who watch it happen
Those who wonder:"What happened?"

Over the last 22 years, I have dedicated hundreds of hours observing the common denominators that make some dental practices very successful, while so many just get by. Members of the more successful dental practices like themselves, enjoy working with each other, and generally have fun! This is not to imply that they do not have their fair share of everyday problems that are experienced by every dental practice in the United States. It simply means that they respond to those problems with a "Take charge and take names attitude." They do not waste time whining or feeling sorry for themselves and measuring the size of the obstacles they encounter until those obstacles become the only things they see. Instead, they seek solutions and answers, and they are firm in their belief that anything is possible and no barriers can prevent them from being the best they can be. The key issue that seems to make a difference is motivation.

Most people, whether in their professional lives or their personal lives, strive for improvement. Wanting change means wanting a change for the better. Wanting change means making a decision to move forward instead of settling for the status quo or sliding backward. The decision is sometimes difficult to make. Though what is out there is attractive, exciting, and inspiring, many of us are afraid of the obstacles that lie between us and the prize. The more we think of the potential obstacles, the more real they become. The more we worry about them, the more insurmountable they become. When we make these obstacles the focus of attention, we diminish that which we want to achieve. Slowly but surely, the prize will recede to ever greater distance; eventually, it will just fade away.

While it is foolish to proceed in life with the false premise that there are no obstacles, it is equally foolish to assume that obstacles are insurmountable. Many of them are nothing more than challenges and opportunities disguised by an ugly face. Approach them with courage and they will shrink proportionately. Motivation will provide the emotional spark needed to find the guts, the strength, character, and commitment that will keep you going when the going gets tough. This applies to personal as well as professional life, and it is important to recognize that how you fare in one area can positively or negatively affect how you fare in the other.

Motivation helps you recognize that there are things you can control and things you cannot control. It helps you understand that the control you exercise over yourself and your reaction to those things beyond your control can make all the difference. Motivation comes from within; it cannot be given to you or taken away from you. It can, however, be practiced and finetuned and perfected until it becomes a way of life. When this happens, obstacles become challenges, things you cannot control become less onerous, and everything you desire becomes possible.

Teaching yourself to be more motivated means making a decision that you would rather be happy than unhappy. It means an attitude adjustment. It means active participation in creating a better professional and personal life for yourself. Sometimes it means taking a chance on yourself. Sometimes it means realizing that there is no disgrace in getting help from someone else. Mostly it means making a commitment to stay upbeat and positive instead of angry, sad, and negative, no matter what the day brings.

While you are restructuring your practice, there will be days that you will wish you had left well enough alone. There may be a day when you wonder why you ever decided to work in the field of dentistry. Prepare for such days by knowing they will come. Do not worry about them in advance and do not worry about them after they have passed.

Maintain positive thinking. Be passionate about your decision. Make sure that you continue to travel in a direction that will make you the best in your field. Practice environment control by surrounding yourself with people who are upbeat and news that is good news. Leave every encounter on a positive note and maintain a sense of humor. Remembering that you have the vision, the goals, the philosophy, and the people needed to make things work is the best motivator of all. You are more than ready to begin the journey of a lifetime.

3 The Pulse of the Pulse of the Practice

In order to succeed in any enterprise, you need to surround yourself with excellent people. When designing your hygiene department, you need to consider very carefully the type of people you want working for you. Whether you are retraining current employees, or hiring new personnel, you can never forget that what happens or doesn't happen in the hygiene department has an impact on the entire dental practice. Your hygienist, for better or worse, will affect patient flow, atmosphere, customer service, marketing, and a host of other things that are critical to the well being of the practice. Someone with this level of responsibility cannot be ordinary or mediocre. The person assuming this position will have enormous responsibilities and must have "star quality"—that special something that can accept the challenge and come up with winning results.

Finding the right dental hygienist means knowing what you need and being willing to pay for it. She must, of course, have excellent clinical skills backed up by a good education. Did she graduate from an accredited institution? Can she answer your questions about commonly used dental products and procedures confidently and accurately? Is she familiar with operatory equipment and technology?

Your candidate should come to the job interview with a degree or certificate from an accredited institution, a transcript that lists the full range of course work and grades, information about internships or prior work experience, and a list of references. These can easily be verified, and a few questions of a clinical nature can provide a general idea of the applicant's clinical knowledge.

Clinical skills, while important, are actually less significant than the candidate's people skills. Training can improve or enhance a hygienist's clinical skills; improving or enhancing personality traits is much more difficult. Assess these carefully by asking the right questions. Why did the applicant choose to enter the dental field? What does she view as an ideal work atmosphere? What features of the job does she enjoy most? Which are most stressful? What skills, besides clinical, does she think she possesses that will help her in performing her duties? What is her position on conflict resolution? How does she feel about working independently? As a member of a team? In what ways does she feel she would contribute to the practice? What, besides a salary, does she expect from the practice?

Interview anxiety is normal and should be expected. At the same time, the way your candidate handles herself during a potentially stressful situation like an interview is a good indicator of how she might perform on a bad day at the office. While interviewing, keep in mind that the hygienist you hire will have to wear many hats. Always consider a working interview. (Fig. 3-1)

Name:_____ Position: _____

Date scheduled: _____

Salary for the day: _____

Duties for the day: _____

Time scheduled   from _____ to _____

Determine if the following skills and attitudes were demonstrated.
Rate the following: (5 represents ideal)

Ability to get along with the team   Job performance
1   2   3   4   5   1   2   3   4   5

Demonstration of excellent clinical skills   Stayed on schedule
1   2   3   4   5   1   2   3   4   5

Degree of difficulty of the day   Positive attitude
1   2   3   4   5   1   2   3   4   5

Professionalism   Appearance
1   2   3   4   5   1   2   3   4   5

List and rate tasks performed: Feedback from your staff:

Second interview or hire? _____

Figure 3–1 The Working Interview

As the staff member who will have the most contact with your patients, the dental hygienist you hire should be able to serve as your most valued goodwill ambassador. If patients respect and trust her, they will respect and trust the practice. Every interaction with a patient is going to be a positive or negative experience that affects patient loyalty, retention, and referrals. Since most patients will spend most of their time in a dental practice with the dental hygienist, she is the one who must bear the heaviest burden of providing customer service that is positive and attractive.

As a representative of your practice, she must be neat, organized, and accurate. She should be a team player who can communicate well with you, other staff members, and especially patients. She must be a good listener, not just a good talker. Good communication is pivotal to a dental practice, and a dental hygienist's ability to communicate is as important as her ability to skillfully perform the clinical tasks required of her. She will be the frontline educator who empowers patients toward a lifetime of ideal dental health. In this capacity, the dental hygienist is the cornerstone of the practice—the one who makes patients decide to come back or stay away. It is her responsibility to make patients aware of their dental problems and to explain the consequences of those problems if they are not treated. If a dental hygienist performs this function effectively, she makes her patients understand and accept the benefits of regular dental care visits. She ensures that patients recognize that a visit to your practice is "not just a cleaning." This instills in patients a good attitude about dental health care and dental health maintenance. If this is done effectively, it can cut the number of "no shows" and significantly raise the number of recare appointments.

Productivity and profit will increase in proportion to the dental hygienist's skill as an educator. This means a commitment to being prepared to answer questions and to project a high level of expertise about dental procedures, dental technology, and dental products. The more she knows, the more she can convey to patients. The more she communicates in a self-confident and knowledgeable manner, the more patients will be willing to listen. The more patients listen and learn, the more they will believe in the benefits of keeping appointments and adhering to a regular dental healthcare schedule in the office and at home.

Job skills should be complemented by people skills. Look for someone with enthusiasm and self-confidence. Look for someone with an interest in self-improvement through continuing education. Never underestimate the importance of loyalty and dedication. You will be entrusting your practice to this person. Choose carefully!

The most important thing to remember before selecting any candidate for the position is a strong code of ethics. According to the preamble of the ADHA Code of Ethics, a dental hygienist is a member of a "community of professionals devoted to the prevention of disease and the promotion and improvement of the public's health." Hygienists are "preventive oral health professionals who provide educational, clinical, and therapeutic services to the public." They "strive to live meaningful, productive, satisfying lives," simultaneously serving themselves, the profession, society, and the world with actions, behaviors, and attitudes that are consistent with a commitment to public service. Use this as a general guideline for selecting the people to whom you will be entrusting your hygiene department and you cannot go wrong.

Hiring pearls

If you are hiring a new person for your hygiene department, you may want to consider a somewhat unorthodox approach to the hiring process. Under the best circumstances, finding someone to fit your needs is difficult. In a lean market, with experienced hygienists and even recent graduates being wooed by practices and institutions willing to pay premium salaries, the task becomes even more daunting.

One way to ease the pain of interviewing scores of wrong applicants before the right one comes along is to begin the "weeding out" process before any applicant walks through the door of the practice. Start with your classified ad. (Fig. 3-2)

> **HELP WANTED**
> Busy dental practice seeks dental hygienist. Minimum three years of experience preferred. Salary negotiable. Call 222-333-4444 for interview.

> **HELP WANTED**
> Excellent dental practice in search of an outstanding dental hygiene professional to manage our non-surgical periodontal and continuing care program. Excellent communication skills are essential. If you want to provide quality care and be appreciated as a professional, please call Cindy at 222-333-4444 for preliminary confidential telephone interview.

Figure 3—2 Classified Ads

The two ads above are radically different. Run the first ad and you will get run-of-the-mill applicants. The experience will be there because you have required it. And you can be reasonably certain that the person responding to this ad will have some clinical skills dictated by the job description. By the same token, you have closed the door to someone with less experience (or no experience) who may have the personal qualities and ambition to become a valuable member of your hygiene department.

The person who responds to the traditional ad will bring the requisite credentials to the interview, expecting and prepared to answer questions about professional competence. Schedules and a salary range may be discussed; references will be checked after the applicant has gone home to wait for a call saying yea or nay. But the person responding to this ad will mostly likely be seeking a "job." In most cases, this applicant will be looking for a job to replace a job already held. If this is the case, it may signal that there is something amiss at the old job.

On the surface, someone who responds to the second ad is a totally unknown quantity. This person may have absolutely no working experience or may have spent summers selling shoes at the mall. She may be extremely competent or woefully lacking in professional skills. She may be leaving another dental practice, but unlike the person responding to the first ad, is not looking for "just a job." No one looking for "just a job" would respond to an advertisement that is so personally slanted. This applicant will be calling because the ad has piqued her interest and has challenged something in her that wants to try something new and exciting and different. Most importantly, this applicant will have enough enthusiasm and guts not to be turned off by the prospect of a "preliminary interview."

Odd as it may seem, a preliminary interview can be conducted over the telephone by you or by a team member who has been with the practice long enough to know what "people qualities" suit the practice dynamics. During this initial phone call, information about previous experience, personal attributes, and communication skills can be elicited. Sample questions might include the following:

1. Where did you go to school?
2. How recently did you graduate?
3. Have you worked as a hygienist before?
4. What job do you presently have?
5. What do you like most about your job?
6. What would you change about your current job?
7. What kind of dentist do you want to work for?

8. What particular skills do you have that would make you good at this job?
9. How much do you think a job like this should pay?
10. Are evenings a problem? Saturdays?

The answers to these questions should provide enough information about the job applicant to determine whether a personal interview is warranted. If the person's responses don't "feel good" to the telephone interviewer, it is more than likely that a personal interview would be a waste of time for everyone concerned.

A strong dental team is essential to the productivity and profitability of the dental hygiene department, and other team members should have something to say about any prospective new hire. Those applicants called back for round two should be interviewed by dental team members, especially by those who will be working in close contact with the new person on a daily basis. Questions should be designed to determine the applicant's feelings about the field of dentistry, about people, and about cooperation in the workplace.

1. Tell us about yourself.
2. Why did you choose to work in the dental field?
3. What kind of work atmosphere would be best for you?
4. What does "team spirit" mean to you?
5. What is your description of an ideal practice?
6. What do you think of people who don't like their jobs?
7. If you had a problem with one of us, what would you do?
8. If you had a problem with your duties in this job, what would you do?
9. If you saw one of us having a problem with a task, what would you do?
10. If you saw one of us having a problem with a patient, what would you do?

An applicant who has answered these questions to the satisfaction of your dental team is certainly worth your attention. Schedule your interview with this person after reviewing her professional and academic credentials. Check educational background and check references. If major irregularities are found in either, you may decide not to proceed with a personal interview at all. If an interview is scheduled, ask questions that will elicit answers about the applicant's attitudes and feelings about supervisors, personal responsibility, patients, continuing education, and professional ethics. Some sample questions follow:

1. How would you handle a patient who frequently misses appointments?
2. What do you expect from this job?
3. Having met the team members, how do you think you will fit in?
4. If you and I don't see eye to eye, how will you try to resolve this?
5. What will you contribute to this position?
6. What will you contribute to this practice?
7. What would you do if your boss made a decision with which you strongly disagree?
8. What would you do if a patient were rude to you?
9. What are your goals in this position?
10. What are your professional goals five years from now? Ten years from now?

There are no guarantees that the person you choose to employ will live up to your expectations. But by designing selection criteria that balance knowledge and skills with wholesome and positive personal characteristics, you definitely improve the odds.

You Get What You Pay For

The laborer is worthy of his hire.
— Luke 10:7

In most practices, staff salaries make up 25–30% of dental overhead. Depending on the size of your hygiene department, up to 11% is hygiene department salary overhead. If you have chosen wisely during the hiring process, do not let these numbers disturb you. Good help *is* hard to find, and is worth paying for. Remember that your hygienists, depending on circumstances you create, can make or break your practice. Ensuring that you get "your money's worth" means having a good financial plan for them. Money talks, and your initial investment should be a commitment to competitive salaries that make your hygienists feel valued and appreciated from the very first day they join your dental team.

Encouraging your hygienists to maintain and improve their skills is also important. This means investing in their continuing education. It means, as well, a commitment to rewarding achievement through an incentive bonus plan. Such a plan challenges them to do their best at all times, to be creative and innovative for the good of the practice. It provides the inspiration for personal and professional success.

Providing a good benefits package is equally important. This includes the obvious—a sound health insurance program—and some less obvious, but equally important perks such as paid holidays, paid vacations, paid personal days, and even paid uniforms.

If you think you cannot afford to pay high salaries, fund continuing education, pay reasonable bonuses, and foot the bill for uniforms, you should take a cold hard look at what can happen if you don't. Master hygienists who are not well compensated, not encouraged to learn new things, and not rewarded for creative and innovative work will not be motivated to do their best. Invariably, they will look beyond the door of your practice for a practice that makes them feel valued, appreciated, and confident. People with these positive qualities and attitudes are happy and productive employees. Happy and productive employees are good for business. Once again, everyone wins.

It is prudent to remember that turnover is the highest overhead expenditure in the dental office. A practice can lose $5,000 to $10,000 in one month's production as a result of losing key personnel. And estimating one month's loss of productivity is just the tip of the iceberg when you consider that it takes about three months to train new people. By providing financial security and financial incentive, you can prevent these and other related problems.

To attract and keep the best, you must be willing to offer the best, and that means offering more than a good salary. Remember that the person you are hiring is not just a tooth picker, but also someone who will contribute many skills and talents to your practice. The right hygienist will not settle for mediocre pay or a ho-hum job. Money, while important, is not the only incentive that attracts good people to a job or profession. Master hygienists want to work in practices that are progressive, organized, and pleasant. Master hygienists are people-oriented and will look for practices where people are valued. Master hygienists ask much of themselves and will look for work that is interesting and challenging. You must provide opportunities for advancement and a pleasant, stable, and safe work environment.

COMMISSION COMPENSATION FOR THE DENTAL HYGIENIST

*Things are only worth what you
make them worth.* —MOLIÈRE

Nationally, 30% to 45% of the gross annual production of a dental practice comes from a properly run recare program. Between 40% and 80% of a dentist's procedures can come from hygiene recare appointments. Up to 75% of all patients should and can be referred to a more frequent recare schedule, and up to 50% should be referred to a more intensive level of periodontal treatment. Less than 10% of patients should be lost through cancellations or broken appointments. In nearly 65% of all practices, orthodontics, cosmetic, and reconstructive dentistry are viewed as extraordinary rather than ordinary procedures.

These numbers are an interesting statistical baseline; in most dental practices they represent a less than optimal level of case acceptance. Unfortunately, in most practices, the preventive maintenance visit or even a periodontal program is seen as an end in itself and is too seldom viewed by hygienists as an opportunity to present optimal dentistry or cosmetic dentistry to patients. Salaries and bonuses notwithstanding, the average hygienist simply may not be motivated nor educated enough to worry about making case acceptance her responsibility.

In a practice with an optimally functioning hygiene department, no one settles for "baseline" or "adequate," but even here, numbers can be improved with a little matter of incentive. So while you are orchestrating changes in your hygiene department, you might want to consider a radically revised view of how a hygienist should be compensated—specifically by looking at the option of introducing a commission program that rewards a hygienist's ability to increase productivity. Hygienists who recommend cross-referenced dentistry to patients and thus improve practice case acceptance of non-periodontal treatments in the practice, expect (and deserve) something more substantial than a congratulatory pat on the back. While there is nothing wrong with merit bonuses, they may be too conservative and traditional for you or your hygienist. Commissions may be an interesting and challenging alternative for both of you.

Establishing commission compensation for your hygiene department requires a mathematical analysis of a hygienist's productivity, potential, and goals. A modest and feasible goal for productivity—say, $700 per day—should be remunerated with a specific commission, roughly in the area of approximately 35%. In real dollar amounts for a three-day week, the hygienist's weekly production of $2,100 would translate to a monthly revenue of approximately $9,000 for the practice. The hygienist's commission compensation for this time period would come to approximately $3,150, or $750 per week.

In calculating case acceptance for each "dentistry seated" appointment, not directly related to hygiene, the commission could be apportioned at a lower percentage, from 5% to 10% of the fee, or at a set dollar amount, ranging from $10 to $50.

Revising pay standards in this manner may be an attractive means of improving departmental and practice productivity and profitability. It is recommended that implementing such a change within your practice be done with the guidance of a trusted consultant, accountant, or attorney.

A Word about Environment

Staffing is critical, but not even the most excellent hygienist can function successfully in the wrong environment. For the hygiene department to be productive and profitable, it must be headquartered in a user-friendly and patient-friendly operatory.

Your hygienist's operatory must be adequately supplied with quality products and equipment. It should be neat, attractive, and comfortable. Supply cabinets should be logically organized; counter space should be orderly and uncluttered. Courtesy packets for patients should be stocked and available for distribution. These might include mouth rinse, toothpaste, toothbrushes, floss, or other incidentals. Wall décor should be professional, but never to the extent that it is intimidating to patients. A light touch, such as a dental comic strip or an amusing mural, is quite acceptable. This is especially true if children visit the practice.

Brochures, charts, posters, booklets, and photographs that will help the hygienist educate patients about oral health conditions, appropriate home care, and restorative or cosmetic procedures should be available in every operatory. A hygienist that has to leave her operatory to rummage in the supply closet for the correct poster is a hygienist who risks losing a patient's interest and attention.

Cleanliness should be strictly enforced. Floors should be spotless; ceilings should be checked for cracked or peeling paint. Always remember that while we are working on a patient's mouth, that patient has nowhere to look but up. A cobweb dangling from that corner is neither attractive nor reassuring. Sinks should be spotless. Disposal bins in the operatory need to be situated so that they are conveniently within the hygienist's reach, but discreetly hidden from patients' view.

Technology should be up-to-date and well maintained. The intraoral camera, the hand-piece equipment, the x-ray machine, the computer terminals, and the light systems should be routinely serviced and properly cared for. Investing in periodic upgrades may be necessary.

Just as important is making certain that the hygienist's comfort is considered. Be aware that one size may not fit all in the operatory. If you have two or more hygienists working in the same space on different schedules, recognize that what is comfortable for one may be extremely uncomfortable for the other(s). A logical, flexible set-up that will accommodate the physical needs of all the hygienists using the space must be jointly decided upon and implemented. A hygiene department cannot function optimally if one hygienist is banging her head on a cabinet and the other is straining muscles to reach something on a shelf that has been improperly hung and inappropriately stocked. Occupational Safety and Health Administration (OSHA) requirements should be strictly adhered to.

SAFETY BEYOND OSHA AND BEYOND HYGIENE

As you work towards your goals of designing and refining an exceptional hygiene department, remind yourself at regular intervals that you are not alone in this new venture—you have a dental team that is pitching in to help! The members of your team may face many of the mixed emotions that keep you awake at night. All of you need to feel that the risk is worth it, and that means installing safety net features for everyone in your practice.

First and foremost, of course, is physical safety for everyone in the practice. OSHA requirements may seem onerous at times, but they are requirements that have arisen from test cases that have proved they are necessary. The health and safety of your practice are possible only if the health and safety of those who work in the practice or visit the practice are assured.

Safety, however, should not be limited to a question of healthy life and limbs. A safe environment for your entire dental team goes beyond OSHA by providing a mental and emotional comfort zone in which team members can work without risk and without chaos. To create such an environment, you need stability. A sane and stable environment can exist only when you, the team leader, provide distinct and clear parameters that everyone on the team understands and adheres to.

Begin with clear definitions. You have already defined the goals and vision of the practice—now you need to make certain that everyone in the practice understands who is responsible for what. It also means letting everyone know that while the hygiene department is the pulse of the practice, every position in the practice is vital and every person in the practice has an important role. This removes the uncertainty that is one of the greatest threats to practice stability.

To bolster these definitions and clarifications, it is crucial to have in place a personnel manual that provides, in black and white, specific criteria about attendance, business conduct, dress code, schedules, benefits, performance ratings, and all other aspects of daily practice life that may be subject to misinterpretation or question.

Grievances of any kind should be dealt with quickly, calmly, and privately. They should never be allowed to fester; they should never become the source of juicy office gossip; they should never, ever, be allowed to interfere with productivity. This leads to chaos and pettiness that undermines office stability and makes the office unsafe and uncomfortable for all.

Safety and security are also dependent on fair and reasonable compensation for all team members. A team member who is worried about keeping the wolf away from the door does not feel safe personally or professionally, and this is sure to have an impact on everyone's productivity.

If everyone associated with the practice is to be truly safe, continuing education is a must. Procedures and products once deemed correct and appropriate may later be recognized as inappropriate and even dangerous. A case in point is mercury-based fillings. Once a professional standard, such fillings have since been discredited from both a dental health and a general health viewpoint.

Make physical, emotional, financial, and mental safety in the practice a priority, and everyone associated with the practice will feel better. Leave these things to chance, and you risk far more than a reprimand from OSHA.

Schedule regular meetings, remembering always that every good meeting has an agenda and that the purpose of each meeting should be constructive, not destructive. Everyone should have a chance to speak, but everyone should also recognize that the objective of any meeting is to resolve issues and problems, not create new ones by turning the meeting into a gripe session. Everyone should feel "safe" when expressing an opinion; everyone should feel "safe" when discussing large or small issues with colleagues and with you.

Unless every person and every department in the practice is safe and stable, your best intentions and most grandiose plans for the hygiene department will fail. (Fig. 3-3)

Punctuality: Be prepared to greet and seat the patient five minutes prior to morning appointment, and after lunch. This means we are waiting for the patient, not making the patient wait for you.

Time: Make every effort to stay within the time frame allotted for each patient by being better organized, better prepared, and being constantly aware of the time. Know something about each patient. Reviewing a patient's record the day before an appointment will allow you to "rehearse" what you are going to say to a patient regarding presentation after treatment.

Educating patients: This is your primary responsibility for every patient. By using pamphlets, brochures, and the intraoral camera, your focus will change from being concerned only about a scale and polish to servicing our patients by presenting dental treatment that best serves them.

Team player: You will begin to think in terms of what *you* can do to better help *your* coworkers by taking *full* responsibility for *your* actions. Your employer has provided you with superior working conditions, instruments, and opportunities to obtain skill and knowledge to fulfill your livelihood as a dental hygienist. Your team players have committed to providing the best of their skill, knowledge, and attitude to provide the atmosphere for you to practice dental hygiene. You will agree to focus, unconditionally, your *attitude* (the wanting to do for others) in the best interest of *your* patients, coworkers, and employer during the hours that you are working.

Accountability: By being accountable for your responsibilities as a dental hygienist, you will begin to have a sense of controlling your own direction. You will be as good as you want to be by your own choice. If you want to develop your skill and knowledge, nobody will stand in your way. If you choose not to develop yourself, it is your own decision. Our practice has made the commitment to make the necessary changes to allow for growth. We want you to make the same commitment.

I, _____fully understand the discussion of these goals and agree to make every effort to utilize them to perform my services as a dental hygienist. This will be reviewed in 30 days.

Employee: _____   Date: _____
Employer: _____   Date: _____

Figure 3–3 Setting Goals to Increase Your Hygienist's Job Performance:
An Agreement Form

4 The Power of Teamwork and Team Spirit

> *Everyone has won and all must have prizes.* — LEWIS CARROLL

As you focus on building and energizing a productive and profitable hygiene department, you can never forget that the pulse of the practice cannot flourish in an environment that is unhealthy and unstable. You can never lose sight of what is going on in the rest of the practice, and you can never neglect what is going on with the rest of your dental team. All of them will contribute to the success of your grand design in direct proportion to the way in which you contribute to their well being. Success depends on everyone, and for this reason, everyone must enjoy professional fulfillment. Making this happen depends on excellent management skills.

In a recent nationwide survey of dental team members, several questions relating to job satisfaction were asked. The responses categorized, tabulated, and analyzed are very revealing. They show a general dissatisfaction with the way things are and pinpoint specific areas that could be and should be addressed by every dental practice.

There is a lack of effective communication between the doctor and the team members

Because a dental team has learned all the ropes and has performed well for a while, many dental practitioners assume that a laissez faire approach to practice management is fine. While a certain amount of autonomy is a good thing, it is important to remember that the practice is *your* practice and that a certain amount of guidance is always needed. Procedures and treatment plans change as technology and medicines change. It is never wise to assume that everyone will get the hang of it sooner or later. Dental teams work best when they are well informed.

The doctor needs to express himself positively instead of being so negative

Evaluate honestly the tone and manner in which you address team members. Do you focus on things that go wrong without commenting on things that are going right? When was the last time you complimented one of your team members on a job well done or even a new haircut? Did you notice that someone took the initiative to finally move the whitening trays, which had been taking up space in a cabinet designated for paper products? Was this person thanked or even acknowledged? What about that missing chart? Was the person who finally found it thanked before you grabbed it and ran to placate the irate patient? How about afterwards? There will be errors and flaws that you should and will comment on, but never forget that there are good things to comment on too.

Office procedures and protocol are not clear or are not consistent

This is partly a problem with communication and partly a problem with haphazard adherence (or no adherence at all) to office policies on assorted matters. These can range from putting away supplies to dress code to effective scheduling that leaves neither patients nor team members sitting around waiting for something to happen. Do you always notice when supply boxes remain unopened on the floor of the coat closet, or is this something that you spot only when a patient can't hang up a jacket because the boxes have been stacked too high? Does the team member who happens to be nearby get criticized or does the whole staff get reamed out? Did the hygienist show up in an inappropriate outfit on Wednesday? Commenting on this is acceptable, but did you also notice that the dental assistant did it the week before? Has the same patient been sitting in the waiting room waiting for a PMV the last three times you have escorted an exiting patient to the door? Are you going to blame the front desk person or the hygienist for this gaff, or are you going to take appropriate steps to fix it?

An appropriate response to all three of the uncomfortable scenarios described above means having an office manual, which specifically outlines what is appropriate and inappropriate policy and protocol in your practice. If you have such a handbook in which these and other potential problems areas are addressed, your team members aren't reading it or may have decided that it doesn't matter because you yourself are not consistent in following the rules and guidelines. Your paper tiger has no bite.

Take the time to reread the office manual with an open eye that sees not only the words on the pages, but their value in real time. The business of dentistry is not inert. Things change, and all changes, whether they come from internal or external forces, must alter policy and protocol accordingly. Make sure that your office manual is not obsolete. If guidelines and information are outdated, update them. If there are too many rules, get rid of those that are petty. *Pay specific attention to how your plans for the hygiene department are going to change old policy and protocol.* Your consultant will guide you in deciding how the policy must change to adhere to the new protocol. Have a wage and labor lawyer review it to make sure it is up to par legally.

If no office handbook exists, it is definitely the time to create one. Do this with the help of team members. You may think you know all the problem areas, but they know things about the practice and about the office that may surprise you and may teach you a thing or two.

Getting team members to work on the manual has other benefits: it will remind team members that there is an office manual, it will encourage active participation in office policy, and it will show all team members that their opinions are valued and respected.

Manual Pearls

Union gives strength. — Aesop

Working with others can be an enjoyable experience or an experience filled with frustration. Each individual in the practice is important, but the team's potential as a well-functioning unit is even more important. If everyone acts responsibly, participates, cooperates, and communicates, everyone benefits. For this to happen, everyone must know what is what. Your office manual should provide the answers to 13 very basic questions:

1. What goes into personnel records?
2. What defines full-time, part-time, over-time, and temporary?
3. What is seniority and how valuable is it?
4. What are my job responsibilities?
5. What is my schedule? What about lunch? What about breaks?
6. What about holidays, vacations, sick leave, personal days, mental health days?
7. What is my role in office safety and security?
8. What is my role in an emergency or crisis?
9. What are the deciding factors that define salary, raises, and bonuses?
10. What are the benefits?
11. What are the guidelines for meetings?
12. What are the guidelines for appearance?
13. What are the guidelines for performance evaluation?

Equally important to the office manual is that it addresses teamwork and practice responsibilities that are not specific to any one position, but specific to the practice philosophy:

1. How you enjoy yourself, your job, your place of work, the dentistry you practice, and your fellow employees is possible to the extent that you make it possible.
2. If you give 100% of yourself to the practice, you will be rewarded in kind.

3. Update your professional skills through continuing education.
4. Be as valuable to the practice as you can be. Complete all work assigned to you. If you finish your assigned tasks early, help someone else.
5. Come to work each day well rested, alert, and properly nourished.
6. Accept responsibility for your actions.
7. Provide your team members with a supportive environment in which they can work and communicate comfortably.
8. Be here because you choose to be here.
9. Practice honesty and integrity.
10. Never hold back the people you work with, and you will feel safe and secure in the knowledge that they will not hold you back.
11. Respect the confidentiality of patients and team members.
12. Support other team members and help them live by these guidelines. They will return the favor.
13. Believe that living by these guidelines is not only polite, but also absolutely critical for effective and meaningful relationships within this practice.

In a setting where management is effective, these guidelines will truly mean something. In a setting where management is *in*effective, they will be as meaningful as the pretty aphorisms on greeting cards—"Gee! What a nice thought!"

For specific information about job descriptions and responsibilities, review Figure 4-1.

Patient Care/Hygiene Coordinator

Job Duties

Goal: Complete responsibility for the organization and profitability of the dental hygiene department

1. Maintain hygiene schedule to daily production goal
2. Confirm appointments with patients
3. Maintain recare system—pre-appoints 100% of recare patients
4. Maintain cancellation, non-appointment list
5. Schedule patients who do not make their 3-, 4-, 5-, or 6-month return visits
6. Responsible for flow of patients
7. Run morning huddle – hygiene section
8. Greet incoming patients
9. Complete chart audits
10. Assist patients with forms, etc.
11. Assist practice with any insurance responsibility
12. Type (and/or) design all correspondence to be utilized with patients
13. Implement acknowledgment system for patient referrals with the help of the entire staff
14. Responsible for screening the hygiene telephone calls
15. Responsible for pulling and filing patients' files
16. Maintain the marketing/customer service program with the hygienists and other staff
17. Maintain departmental statistics and be able to evaluate the health of the department
18. Facilitate the monthly departmental meeting
19. Electronic claims submission
20. Collection over the counter, if necessary
21. O.H.I., if necessary
22. Treatment presenting

Additional Duties: Assist with clinical responsibilities (usually seen with a multiple hygiene department)

Radiograph updates

Charting

Operatory turnover

Medicament instruction

Sterilization

Medical history updates

Assisting with periodontal probing

Figure 4–1 Job Descriptions and Responsibilities

Front Desk Coordinator

Job Duties

Goal: Complete accountability to ensure a productive and profitable dental practice

1. Front desk and reception are kept clean and neat for all to see
2. Patients greeted promptly by name as they enter office/alert doctor(s) and hygienist(s) when patient(s) arrive
3. Referrals tracked/thank you's sent
4. Copy made of schedule for each operatory (including TX amounts for each patient and total for the day)
5. Routing slips or treatment cards put with each chart
6. Treatment entered on computer and appropriate statement printed efficiently and accurately
7. Control inventory of office supplies and forms
8. Knowledge of treatment procedure sequence
9. Reinforcing patient comfort
10. Follow up on patient, insurance company, or other dentists' requests
11. Accurately complete and use all patient file documents
12. Call patients seen, if the doctor needs to have them called
13. Confirm appointments with appropriate lead-time
14. Documents broken and failed appointments
15. Maintain call list via computer and list cards to fill change in schedule
16. Pre-appoint recares if not done by hygiene department
17. Engineer the schedule (including scheduling)
18. Takes initiative in collecting each fee/co-payment at the time of service
19. Inform patient of financial policy at initial visit and in the course of treatment
20. Monitor and reports monthly the AR informing doctor of status and problems
21. Follow-up on payment problems in a timely manner and with specific collection procedure
22. Bank deposits made accurately and in a timely manner
23. Insurance forms properly completed and appropriate radiographs enclosed for processing/follow-up overdue insurance claims/payments
24. Provide valuable internal marketing for practice via patient contact
25. Post all personal payments and insurance payouts
26. Make sure that daily sheet balances
27. Do electronic claims and run reports
28. Keep appointment book or computer scheduler
29. Keep schedule for doctor's meetings
30. Facilitate appropriate meetings

Figure 4–1 continued

Dental Assistant

Job Duties

Goal: To maintain excellence in the clinical area of the dental practice

1. Operatory clean and neat before patient seating
2. Greet and seat patient
3. Update medical history
4. Have instruments readily available for procedure and provider
5. Chart accurately
6. Complete patient records (i.e., treatment cards, front desk sheet, make sure radiographs are with chart)
7. Proficient with sequence of all dental procedures
8. Reinforce patient comfort
9. Patient education
10. Post-op instructions
11. Take alginate impressions
12. Pour impressions, trim and clean molds
13. Lab cleanliness
14. Restock operatory supplies (including tubs)
15. Wipe down operatory and clean light
16. Proper sterilization techniques (i.e., bag instruments correctly)
17. Perform excellent clinical techniques chair side with doctor
18. Maintain consistent C.E. schedule
19. Run autoclave periodically throughout the day
20. Proficient with radiograph procedures
21. Bag excess garbage
22. Clean suction
23. Change ultrasonic solution
24. Turn off vacuum, master switch, x-ray, film processor, music, lights
25. Participate in team/departmental meetings
26. Is always a team player
27. Excel in customer service

Figure 4–1 continued

Dental Hygienist

Job Duties

Goal: To become the best hygienist in charge of the "Preventive, Periodontal Practice of Care"

1. Complete a comprehensive exam at least once a year—co-assess with the dentist
2. Accurate charting of hard and soft tissue (i.e., decay, periodontal probing, recession, pocket depth, and mobility)
3. Update medical/dental history
4. Discuss appropriate treatment needs. The dentist and hygienist co-assess and confirm recommended treatment. Hygienist educates patient regarding crowns, bridges, root planing, etc.
5. Periodontal conditions evaluated and discussed: closure is completed by the hygienist
6. Complete patient records (i.e., treatment forms, front desk sheet, make sure radiographs are with chart)
7. Excellent clinical skills performed on each patient
8. Hygienist excels in customer service skills
9. Post-op procedures discussed
10. Dental prophylaxis efficiency for children and adults (i.e., removal of deposits, accretions, and stains from surfaces of the teeth and restorations and polishing of the same)
11. Develop and implement a progressive periodontal program
12. Fluoride therapy
13. Oral hygiene program maintained
14. Pit and fissure sealant placement efficiency
15. Thorough and accurate charting of procedure, patient/doctor communication, recommendations, and patient response
16. Proper sterilization techniques
17. Proficiency with radiographic procedures
18. Keep operative neat and orderly
19. Sharpening of instruments
20. Maintain hygiene supplies
21. Maintain patient recare in computer
22. Maintain recare system (including calling or writing patients if necessary)
23. Design and maintain proper hygiene monitors
24. Design schedule for hygiene
25. Maintain set goal for hygiene production

Figure 4–1 continued

MANAGEMENT PEARLS

The buck stops here.
— HARRY S TRUMAN

You and your dental team are in the business of dentistry. This means a twofold responsibility—caring for patients and caring for the practice. Your success in providing excellent dental care to your patients cannot be separated from an uncompromising commitment to the practice. For this reason, all members of the practice need to adhere to a code of ethical and moral guidelines that promotes harmony and solidarity. Anything less leaves the door wide open for stress, hostility, chaos, and failure. Your entire team must understand that working together well truly means doing unto others as you would have them do unto you. It often means being your teammates' keeper. It sometimes means helping others help themselves. And it always means a full commitment to doing what is right, even when doing what is right seems difficult or unfair or tedious.

No business can thrive and grow and prosper when the people involved in the day-to-day functions of that business view it as the place they put in their time just to get a paycheck. If you have even the slightest suspicion that any team member in your practice feels this way, corrective measures need to be implemented as soon as possible. They begin with an honest evaluation of your practice management approach, personnel dynamics within the practice, the practice infrastructure, and your own attitude about your profession, your staff, your patients, and your work.

Set the culture

Begin by recognizing that each person's job is important or it wouldn't exist. That makes every member of your team important. If your team members recognize that you value them and their contributions, they are likely to value themselves and their contributions too. Good practice attitude begins at the top. Individuals who are treated with respect will be more likely to treat others with respect.

Encourage communication and creativity

Remember that communication is a two-way street. The best way to keep traffic moving in both directions is to know when to speak and when to listen. Your team members are intimately involved with your practice and may have some very good ideas about how to improve it. Be open to their ideas even if they come from unexpected sources. Ideas are migratory and they often flourish in new contexts. If you compartmentalize people and their ideas, you may lose valuable insights. The next time the front desk person has a suggestion about storing supplies or trying a new treatment plan on Mrs. Jones, take the time to really listen.

Show appreciation

Happy dental teams consist of individuals who, like all of us, like to be appreciated for the things they do. Thank people. Validate people. Compliment people. Pay people what they deserve to be paid. Wages should reward productivity. Bonuses should not be limited to those year-end checks everybody expects anyway; they should be a reflection of special achievements and accomplishments, awarded to individuals or departments with a note expressing your delight that something was improved or implemented or eliminated or initiated.

Stand by your man (or woman)

People need to know that you support decisions they make, especially if those decisions are based on a sincere effort to evaluate and interpret information that is available to them. If the decision is sound, it should be acknowledged and praised. If the decision shows a less than perfect judgment call, review it for any merits it may have rather than simply trashing it. If the decision is the result of lack of knowledge, point the team member to the correct information. Some decisions made by team members may show a degree of carelessness. Responding to such decisions positively may require a tremendous amount of self-discipline on your part, but it will eventually yield the dividend you want—someone who learns to be more careful and more precise because this is encouraged and expected.

Make all criticism constructive criticism

Practice morale is more important than you may realize. People know when they have or haven't performed well. If team members see that your response to mistakes is constructive, they will be more receptive to your recommendations and advice. Focus on prevention of future mistakes rather than on belaboring the gravity of a mistake that has occurred. Recognize that verbal abuse, no matter how great the provocation, is always counterproductive. Berating a team member, especially in front of other team members or patients, has no positive effect and can permanently damage the relationship you have with that team member.

Be a buffer

Every business in which individuals come together to work together has the potential for stress and for personality conflict. Effective managers encourage an atmosphere where real problems can be faced squarely because petty problems are addressed and dealt with quickly, efficiently, and terminally. In a well-run practice, buffers make sure molehills remain molehills because they recognize that people have enough difficulty dealing with real crises.

Have meetings

One way to make sure that all team members are kept informed is to schedule routine meetings. Meet with members of your staff one to one. Meet with specific departments. Meet with the entire dental team. Find out what is unknown or misunderstood. Find out what the misconceptions are and address them. Let your entire staff know what your expectations are, especially if those expectations have changed in recent months. Find out what their expectations are too. Are there difficulties they do not know how to handle? Are there questions about treatment plans, about equipment, about new products that have been introduced to the practice?

Err on the side of macro-, not micro-management

Give people increasing amounts of latitude as they prove they can live up to your trust in them. Allowing a degree of autonomy leads to creativity and resourcefulness. People who are allowed to be creative and resourceful enjoy their work. People who enjoy their work are more productive and more passionate about their work. Productivity combined with passion equals profitability. This is an unbeatable equation.

Provide guidelines

A dental team "code of ethics" to which everyone subscribes provides basic guidelines. (Fig. 4-2)

Dental Team Code of Ethics

We are committed to the profession we serve and we hold ourselves accountable to high ethical standards in our dealings with our patients and with each other. As members of a practice dedicated to providing ethical treatment and ethical counsel to our patients, we shall:

- Recognize that ethical practices guide us in making informed ethical decisions
- Establish and maintain standards for ethical judgement and conduct
- Expect the highest level of excellence from each team member
- Develop and adhere to written guidelines that express our expectations of ethical behavior
- Provide services reflecting only the highest levels of professional knowledge, judgement, and skill
- Serve as advocates committed to our patients' well-being by providing them with information necessary to make informed decisions about their oral health
- Provide other team members with the information necessary to make informed decisions about their work with patients and with each other
- Encourage our patients and our team members to become partners in achieving optimal oral health
- Keep all professional communication and relationships with patients confidential
- Keep all professional communication and relationships with patients and with each other respectful
- Participate in the advancement of our profession by learning, by teaching, and by exemplary behavior

We hold these principles and general laws of conduct as the foundation of our ethics and as concepts that are to be applied to our profession and our relationships with others at all times.

Figure 4–2 Dental Team Code of Ethics

PROFESSIONAL FULFILLMENT: THE IDEAL PRACTICE POSITION

*Far and away the best prize that
life affords is the chance to work
hard at work worth doing.*
— THEODORE ROOSEVELT

What follows is a list of the ingredients that can make every position in a dental practice a fulfilling one. Please note that these are not ranked in any particular order.

- When taking a personality test, most dental employees rank highest in the area of "influencing others." They are very people-oriented. Your team members chose dentistry because of the people they come in contact with every day. Make sure their workload is always interesting and challenging.
- Employees should feel they are important as individuals. The top 20% dental practices know that in today's dental environment there is a "lateral level of leadership." Everyone is important to the team, and the team makes up the well-oiled gestalt called a practice. Each team member should take charge of his or her area of expertise. All team members should be accountable to each other. Each member must also lead by example.
- Feedback on performance is provided. It is good business to periodically sit down with the team and complete what is called a "personal, professional interview." The purpose of this meeting is to communicate and explore all strengths, weaknesses, and concerns. Remember that viewing the meeting as a "growth appraisal" is more beneficial than viewing it as a reason to carp and criticize. (Fig.4-3)

Employee _____	Ratings:

Ratings:
1. needs major improvement
2. needs minor improvement
3. average
4. does procedures very well
5. excels in area

Date _____

Job description _____

Ability to listen	1	2	3	4	5
Ability to keep personal affairs under control	1	2	3	4	5
Accuracy	1	2	3	4	5
Adaptability	1	2	3	4	5
Attitudes of optimism	1	2	3	4	5
Attitudes of self giving	1	2	3	4	5
Cooperation with co-workers	1	2	3	4	5
Cooperation with employer	1	2	3	4	5
Cooperation with patients	1	2	3	4	5
Daily attendance (punctuality)	1	2	3	4	5
Dependability, follow through	1	2	3	4	5
Diplomacy and tact	1	2	3	4	5
Establishes and achieves high standard of performance	1	2	3	4	5
Establishes meaningful relationship with patient	1	2	3	4	5
Genuine, active love for people	1	2	3	4	5
Initiative	1	2	3	4	5
Knowledge of job	1	2	3	4	5
Manages time efficiently	1	2	3	4	5
Markets internally	1	2	3	4	5
Markets externally	1	2	3	4	5
Masters communicative skills	1	2	3	4	5
Memorizes and studies schedule	1	2	3	4	5
Personal appearance	1	2	3	4	5
Personality	1	2	3	4	5
Willingly accepts suggestions and constructive criticism	1	2	3	4	5
Willingly volunteers to assist other staff members	1	2	3	4	5

Primary functions (in order of importance)

_____ 1 2 3 4 5
_____ 1 2 3 4 5
_____ 1 2 3 4 5

Growth since last review 1 2 3 4 5

Figure 4–3 Growth Appraisal

- Rewards are strongly related to performance. The most fundamental management principle states, "What gets rewarded, gets done." It is just human nature to look forward to something. Remember that rewards come in all shapes and sizes. A program that rewards its team members for a job well done will always produce a happy, motivated team.

- A good team is good at setting goals. Direction is really all that the motivated, organized team needs. The team will list the priorities that must be accomplished to reach each goal. (Fig. 4-4)

EMPLOYEE PERFORMANCE APPRAISAL/DENTAL HYGIENE

Employee name _____

Date _____ **Appraisal period** _____

General Instructions

The employee performance appraisal is based on the following factors:
1. The employee's dependability and dedication to the team and team goals; and
2. The employee's level of proficiency in executing job duties.

Levels of Achievement

Unacceptable (0)	Improvement needed (1)	Effective (2)
Failed to demonstrate adequate progress toward completion of goals/responsibilities. Did not demonstrate skills & knowledge.	Accomplished some but not all goals and/or responsibilities. Skills & knowledge could be used more effectively.	Accomplished goals and/or responsibilities. Productively utilized skills & knowledge to perform job.

Highly effective (3)	Outstanding (4)
Accomplished goals and/or responsibilities beyond expectations. Commendably used skills & knowledge to excel on job.	Consistently exceeded goals and/or responsibilities. Shows overall excellence in skills & knowledge.

Figure 4–4 Employee Performance Appraisal/Dental Hygiene

For each performance standard, evaluate the level of achievement demonstrated by the Employee during the review period.

Performance Standards	Level of Achievement
1. Cooperation/team effectiveness: Works effectively with others toward team goals. Contributes to morale and teamwork.	
2. Dependability: Demonstrates reliability in attendance and timeliness of work. Meets deadlines.	
3. Flexibility/adaptability: Adjusts behavior, style, or schedule as situation requires. Handles multiple tasks.	
4. Independence: Performs work assignments with minimum need for supervision. Looks for ways to contribute.	
5. Interpersonal skills: Creates climate of open communication and courtesy toward others. Listens attentively and respects privacy and confidentiality.	
6. Job knowledge: Possesses skills and technical competence to execute job duties and operate within office policies, procedures, and safety standards.	
7. Management support: Keeps supervisor well informed and responds positively to job requests and leadership of supervisor.	
8. Productivity/time management: Demonstrates ability to set priorities, establish limits, and achieve results. Schedules and uses time efficiently.	
9. Responsibility/commitment: Dedicates effort, resources, and time to get the job done in cost-effective manner. Dresses and acts professionally and appropriately.	
10. Problem solving: Identifies problem areas and secures data or assistance to resolve them.	
11. Communication: Uses appropriate language and grammar when speaking or writing. Is sensitive to others' concerns and needs for dignity and respect.	

Figure 4–4 continued

Ratings For Specific Job Duties
(where applicable)

Job Duty	Rating	Job Duty	Rating
Pursues continuing education courses to improve skills		Pit and fissure sealant placement accuracy	
Examines hard & soft tissue carefully		Proper sterilization techniques	
Accurate charting of hard & soft tissue		Stays on schedule	
Updates medical history properly		Proficiency with radiographic procedures	
Thorough & accurate charting of procedures		Ability to handle patient problems & questions	
Periodontal condition evaluated & discussed		Keeps operatory neat and orderly	
Discusses appropriate treatment needs		Sharpens instruments correctly	
Post-op procedures discussed		Maintains patients recare notes & system	
Dental prophylaxis is efficiently completed on all patients		Provides internal marketing	
Gentleness in treatment of patients		Pre-appoints the patients	
Excellent root planing and scaling skills		Promotes the practice	
Completes proper fluoride therapy		Refers to the practice	
Communication to doctor, communicates findings			
Excellent educational skills			
Offers support to team when needed			

Figure 4–4 continued

- Passion. It is essential that passion be a visible and constant factor in the practice. Every team member should feel passion for the practice as well as for his or her individual position in that practice. Good attitude, compassion, and confidence will follow naturally and resoundingly.
- Opportunity for advancement. Advancement in dentistry can be almost impossible if you don't continue to improve your level of academic education. However, through on-the-job training, every team member can move into other management areas within the practice. For example, the hygienist can take responsibility for the whitening program. An assistant can develop a nutritional counseling program for the patients.
- Getting along with the team. A successful person must feel like part of a loving "family" in the dental office. Since we spend the longest

part of our day with co-workers, it is important to get along with everyone most of the time.

- Having a management team that avoids "crisis management." Putting out fires is not fun, nor does it help to improve the practice over time. Meeting obstacles head on by scheduling monthly department meetings is good preventive strategy. Overcome the problems and put on paper a plan of action that will keep you moving ahead in the appropriate direction.
- Having management that appreciates its employees.

Always give people more than they expect and the rewards of success will always be yours!

For any problems that may be brought up, commit a list of solutions to paper. (Fig. 4-5)

1. Review the vision, mission, and goals for the practice.
2. Are we reaching and exceeding the goals each month? If not, why not?
3. List the barriers that exist which keep us from reaching the goals.
   - Administration
   - Dental assisting
   - Hygiene
   - Doctor
4. List all the possible solutions to each of the barriers as shared in #3.
5. Create the action plan to implement the solutions.

   Deadline dates:

   Who will be involved:

Figure 4–5 Practice Growth and Success

Attitude Pearls

*They can do all because they think
they can. – Virgil*

Someone once said to me that what I will become in five years will depend on the books I read, the television I watch, the movies I see, and the people I hang around with. Everyone knows that we have a tendency not to want to be around negative people. Instead, we are automatically drawn to people who are positive, upbeat, and self-confident. The following are priority items that you and your team members should put into place daily, weekly, monthly, and annually.

Choose to have a positive attitude

Always present a warm, positive outlook on life. We have all heard the expression, "When life throws you a lemon, make lemonade!" It is a conscious effort to replace negative, self-defeating thoughts with positive self-fulfilling thoughts. It takes hard work, determination, enthusiasm, and self-control to be positive. Develop self-control.

Build an appreciation of yourself

Enjoy and be satisfied with your own uniqueness. List your strengths and weaknesses. Are there strengths buried in those weakness? How can you turn them around to make them strengths? How will this help you to reach your potential?

Show only a positive personality

Never speak of anyone or anything in a negative way. Praise others and show appreciation. Be a giver, not a taker.

Learn from your defeat

Every failure carries with it an opportunity to improve the next time. "Learn from your mistakes!" If something doesn't work, figure out why and change it. We either grow from our mistakes or we become victims.

Trust your own judgment

Believe in yourself.

Share your success

Remember that when others know of your plans, they will encourage and support you. People like to be around positive people because positive people are winners!

Do it now

Never put off till tomorrow what you can do today.

5 Meetings

THE REASON FOR MEETINGS

We are taught early on in our careers that a dental practice is a business. All team members need to embrace this reality. All must master the principles that empower the business. This means listening to the customers, fostering effective communication between the boss and the employees, training, helping, and supporting each other, and monitoring the health of the business on a daily, monthly, and annual basis.

With so many internal and external factors affecting the health of the dental team and the practice, it is necessary to take time to communicate concerns, list obstacles that stand in the way of success, and talk about what must be done to overcome these obstacles. This "quality" time is called the meeting. We cannot excel in the business of dentistry unless we take the time to set goals, establish priorities, and solve problems in a way that coordinates efforts and ideas. Meetings allow us to accomplish this on an ongoing basis.

In a practice with the hygiene department at its core, productive meetings are especially important because hygiene problems, hygiene productivity, and hygiene profitability are everybody's business.

MEETINGS THAT DON'T WORK

It has been noted by some experts in dental management that well conducted, *productive* meetings held once or twice a month for about two hours can increase practice revenues by almost 30%. Please note that the word productive is stressed here. Most meetings held by average dental practices are not productive.

Almost universally, meetings have become complaint sessions as staff members think that a meeting agenda focuses on griping about how bad things are. Almost universally, meetings are chaotic and unfocused, because no one has taken the time to create an orderly agenda. Almost universally, meetings are boring and resented as a waste of time, because most become a pulpit for a long-winded lecture from somebody, and most of the information discussed seems to have no relevance to anything.

A recent poll of more than 500 dental team members listed the following as the 10 most common reasons meetings fail:

1. Lack of leadership/facilitation
2. Failure to keep open minds
3. Hesitancy to be candid and express viewpoints that may be controversial
4. Fear of taking risks, or making changes that lead only to safe solutions and outcomes
5. Coworkers become bored and attention wanders
6. One person dominates the discussion
7. Coworkers engage in side conversation
8. Meetings drag on and on and on
9. Coworkers are not focused because an agenda was not prepared
10. Everyone takes the safest route by reaching decisions that will please the most people

It is small comfort that meetings in other businesses suffer from the same ailment. In too many cases, meetings are scheduled for the sole reason that conventional business wisdom dictates that they should happen every now and again. Unfortunately, the one part of the conventional business that seems to be ignored is that bad meetings are worse than no meetings. And most meetings, as we have all observed, are bad meetings.

It is critical to remember that unproductive meetings are also costly. The master dental practice invests almost 9% of its in-office production time scheduling and having meetings. The average cost to schedule and have teams participate in meetings ranges from $300 to $1,000 per hour. Calculating how much is wasted annually on unproductive meetings is the best incentive for change.

MEETINGS THAT DO WORK

There is a way to do it better. Find it.
— THOMAS ALVA EDISON

Making meetings productive begins with setting policy. Meetings should become part of the practice routine. They should not happen "sometime this month." There should be a regular schedule and a focused agenda. The regularity and structure of team meetings allow for continuous, consistent communication, which keeps the team focused on practice direction.

It is important to incorporate meeting protocol into your office manual. The most important components are frequency, attendance, and purpose. Everyone has a role to play.

SOME MEETING GROUND RULES

Frequency and purpose. Team meetings will be held twice a month, for two hours. One of these meetings will focus on a continuing educational presentation by an assigned team member. The other meeting's topic will be on the business of the practice. Department meetings will be held once a month. A morning huddle will be held every business day. A practice retreat will be held once a year.

Who needs to show. Attendance at meetings is required. If a team or departmental meeting is held on an employee's regular day off, the employee will be paid the regular salary rate for time spent at the meeting, unless overtime is appropriate. If a meeting is missed, the employee is responsible for reviewing what was covered at the meeting. A memo of what transpired should be left in the employee's mailbox.

People. All meetings will have a *facilitator*, a person in charge. This position can be rotated among team members or department members. The facilitator produces an agenda and provides a copy of the agenda for everyone attending the meeting. She makes sure the meeting starts and stops on time. She keeps the focus on the agenda and prevents other participants from becoming bogged down on any single item. She also has the responsibility of keeping the meeting positive and squashing whining before it gets a chance to proliferate. The facilitator records proceedings and makes sure that everyone receives a copy of the minutes. A loose-leaf binder with notes of all meetings should be consistently maintained. Typed copies of minutes should be left in each team member's mailbox. Team and department *members* should come to meetings prepared to participate. Everyone should present topics for discussion to the facilitator before the meeting. The *doctor* should set the parameters or detail any necessary criteria and then step back into the role of team member. The one caveat in this is that the doctor has *veto* power.

Agendas. Team and departmental meetings will follow clearly established rules and agendas. Any agenda items not discussed are referred as priority for the next agenda. The topics should be introduced as old business/priority. This way everyone will know that the concerns they had during the last meeting are of value and will be covered.

Nothing makes a meeting more productive than a solid and focused agenda. Figures 5-1 through 5-6 are a few good models that can be tailored to suit your specific practice needs.

Date: _____   **Practice:** _____

Practice Health Reports:

Production – MTD _____   Collection - MTD _____

New patients_____   Hygiene report _____

Dental assisting report _____   Administration _____

Old Business: (list need-to-be-reviewed items)

Item 1 _____

_____

_____

Item 2 _____

_____

_____

Item 3 _____

_____

_____

New Business: (new agenda items)

Item 1 _____

_____

_____

Item 2 _____

_____

_____

Item 3 _____

_____

_____

Content Discussion: (usually a clinical C.E. presentation; can be assigned to certain team members to present.)

Next meeting date: _____

Facilitator:_____

Recorder: _____

Topics to discuss: _____

Figure 5–1 Team Meeting Agenda (once a month for two hours)

Date: _____

I. Financial report: _____
_____
_____

II. Announcements: _____
_____
_____

III. Review of commitment from last staff meeting: _____
_____
_____

IV. Department Reports
Business office: _____
_____

Chair-side assistants/lab: _____
_____

Hygiene department: _____
_____

Doctor: _____
_____

V. Discussion of posted topics, concerns, reminders, new ideas, and suggestions:
_____
_____

VI. Strategic planning and GOAL setting for next month: _____
_____
_____

VII. Individual commitments to be accomplished by the next meeting: _____
_____
_____

Figure 5–2 Staff Meeting Agenda

Date: _____ **Leader:** _____
Recorder: _____

Content: Creating an ideal hygiene department

Review Philosophy of Practice. This should be written up and staff should agree to the mission statement and work to achieve its goals.

Review Vision. Doctor shares in the direction the practice is headed. The vision includes long-range goals.

List any barriers that could keep us from attaining the vision.

Set Goals for the Department. Remember that one hygienist can produce $1,000-$1,200 or more each day.

Begin the Development of the Dental Hygiene Program.
Define what is a prophylaxis style of patient.
Discuss how new patients will be handled.
Discuss how we will begin to diagnose disease.
Begin the written policy for the periodontal patient and how to implement.
(Please refer to all of the enclosed forms, letters, etc. that I have provided to you)
Scheduling protocol
Treatment planning scripts and communication
Marketing action plan
Other

Commitments: _____ **Deadline:** _____
Next Meeting: _____
Topic: _____

Figure 5–3 Hygiene Meeting Agenda

Bring the Following:
- Reports
- Numbers
- Monitors
- Goal

I. Numbers month-to-date.
II. What's not working? What needs improving?
III. What is working? Make a list of positive things.
IV. Report of department.
V. Personal, Professional Review:
- Why do you work?
- Why do you work here?
- What can you do to improve and create a more positive work environment?
- What can I do to improve and create a more positive work environment?
VI. Review of goals, vision, etc.
VII. Other:

Figure 5–4 Departmental Meeting Agenda (1)

Review of Mission and Goals for the Department
Review of current month-to-date numbers
Are we under or over in respect to our goals?
Pearls. Please share any clinical or management ideas with the group.

Content Discussion:
- What are the major weaknesses of our department?
- What are the major strengths in our department?
- Prepare three creative solutions to the weak areas.
- Decide how to implement the solutions and who will be accountable.

Case Presentation. Each hygienist will report her monthly numbers.
How can we improve our ability to get patients to say, "yes" to better or more ideal dentistry?

Production. Each hygienist will report her monthly numbers.

Review Ideal Days. Number of case starts for periodontal, radiograph review, customer service strategies, etc.

Goals until Next Meeting:

Meeting Date, Facilitator, Recorder, etc.

Content Discussion:

Please type notes and be sure to pass out a copy to each staff member.
Don't forget to schedule deadline dates.
Are you going to attend any continuing education courses?

Figure 5–5 Departmental Meeting Agenda (2)

Review Mission Statement/Purpose of Practice

Review Goals of the Department

Month-to-date Numbers. Where are we positioned at this time?

Review of Previous Meeting Notes.
- Have we completed the objectives from the previous meeting?
- How is our department doing now?
- Are there any weaknesses/barriers affecting us now?
- List the solutions to these weaknesses/barriers.
- Which will be implemented within the next 30 days?
- Who's responsible?
- List the deadline date:
- Are we continuing to follow up?
- Set the dates to follow up on consistency.

List the Strengths of the Department.

Final Notes and Thoughts:

Next Meeting:
Date: _____
Topic: _____
Facilitator: _____
Recorder: _____

Members Present:

Figure 5–6 Departmental Meeting Agenda (3)

The Morning Huddle: Making Every Day a Great Day

During a football game, the coach calls for a huddle during which players quickly psyche themselves and review the strategy for the next play. In a dental practice, a 10-minute morning huddle allows us to anticipate problems that may arise and concentrate on proactive solutions that will smooth the rough spots and eliminate stress. The morning huddle is extremely important for the well being of every practice because it accentuates the fact that daily production is a part of the yearly goal. Because we can control annual production only one day at a time, we need to make each day count. When working well for a practice, the morning huddle will increase production as much at 25%.

You must adhere to some strict management guidelines when orchestrating the morning huddle:

- Everyone should be present
- Set and maintain a positive tone
- Begin promptly and end promptly
- Make sure the huddle is not interrupted
- Check answering machine before morning huddle
- Have a written agenda to follow
- Come prepared with charts, schedules, and appointment books
- Remain standing—the huddle is meant to move very fast so there is no time to become comfortable
- Don't tolerate "Front doesn't understand the back, and the back does not understand the front—don't tolerate negativity"
- Don't tolerate a huddle that turns into a story-telling session

Though every practice should set specific criteria for its morning huddle agenda, three important components should take top billing.

1. **Numbers** define practice productivity and should be addressed at every morning huddle. Review yesterday's productivity. Check today's overall production schedule and hygiene production schedule. Review month-to-date productivity and assess whether goals are being met. How many patients were seen yesterday? How many patients are being seen today? How many patients are due for x-rays? How many patients started or completed STM periodontal programs? Did we have emergency patients yesterday? New patients today? Referrals?

2. **Dollars** define practice profitability. Review yesterday's collections and month-to-date collections and assess whether goals are being met. What are dollar amounts of treatment plans presented yesterday? Dollar amounts of treatment plans accepted by patients yesterday? Is the ratio acceptable? If not, what should be corrected? Review financial arrangements made yesterday and those projected for today's patients.

3. **Scheduling** determines both productivity and profitability. Check telephone messages before the morning huddle to see if any of the messages will affect the day's schedule. If someone has canceled, can someone else be called for an appointment? If someone wants an emergency appointment, what is the best time to have that person come in? If someone on the team has down time, can that person help smooth things for another department or for the practice in general?

Postscript. Look at the entire schedule. Is this a good week? If not, what would you change about it? After any messages received today or any schedule changes, what are you left with? How can you save today's schedule? Is there enough information in the sample appointment book to quickly evaluate the schedule? What should be routinely included with each entry made?

Before ending the morning huddle, ask team members what can be done to make the day better. Always end the morning huddle on a positive note. Remind team members they are terrific and they will be happy to prove it to you.

Figures 5-7 and 5-8 offer samples of morning huddle agendas that you can adopt for your own practice.

1. Is today going to work? _____ Changes:_____
2. M-T-D Production _____ Above or below goal? _____
3. M-T-D Collection _____ Above or below goal? _____
4. Today's doctor production: _____ Goal: _____
5. Today's hygiene production:_____ Goal: _____
6. Names of patients who are overdue for x-rays or hygiene.
7. What patients are candidates for periodontal programs today?
8. Review of patients who still need to be treatment planned/presented.
9. Review of financial arrangements for today's patients.
10. Review today's new patients. Referral source?
11. Where should emergency patients be placed in the schedule?
12. If there are cancellations, what can we do to help each other?

Figure 5-7 Morning Huddle Agenda (1)

Today M-T-D
- Production numbers – MTD - practice
- Collection numbers- MTD - practice
- Are we reaching and exceeding our goals? If not, why not?

Doctor: Is today going to work?
- Are goals going to be reached? If not, how can we improve?
- Where do you want emergencies?
- Highlight new patients
- Personal information on the patients

Organize flow of patients with the team. Will we be on time?
If opening in schedule, what can I do to assist the rest of the team?

Hygiene: Is today going to work? Scheduling and time?
- Month to date report – production – health statistics
- Will I reach my goals today? If not, why not?
- Review patient files and treatment planned in the schedule
- Will I need to update on the patients:
  1. Personal information
  2. Radiographs
  3. Periodontal probing
  4. Comprehensive medical review
  5. Treatment not yet accepted

If there is an opening, do we know of anyone to call?

Figure 5–8 Morning Huddle Agenda (2)

ANNUAL RETREATS

We have already established that holding productive staff meetings is an important element of dental business and that unproductive meetings are useless and costly. For this reason alone, it is very wise to make sure that the meetings are organized, motivating, and result-oriented.

This cannot happen if *purpose and content* are not provided to the participants before the meeting. If the team does not know why a meeting has been scheduled, they might not be prepared to provide information that would be relevant and useful. If they haven't thought about the issues beforehand, then their thoughts won't be as well articulated. If they don't know the meeting's agenda, they can't help each other stick to it, and the meeting will get off track.

An especially good annual investment is an office retreat where purpose and content are highlighted for a review of the preceding year and for creating or amending a vision for the year to come. The meeting should take one whole day and should be held offsite. Impress upon all concerned that the purpose of the meeting is business-oriented and not just a day in the country.

As always, for the meeting to be effective, a leader, moderator, or facilitator must be in charge. Unless you have a specific reason for doing otherwise, always let meeting participants know the following information beforehand.

Date, place and time

Since everyone will be expected to participate, make certain that this information is provided well in advance so that all team members can make plans accordingly. Remind everyone that patients should not be scheduled for the day of the retreat. Give a definitive starting time and stopping time, building in appropriate slots for meals and breaks.

Purpose and content

Define the purpose of the meeting, specifying exactly what you want to accomplish. Prepare the agenda and pass out copies approximately one to two weeks before the scheduled date of the meeting. List results expected from the meeting. These should be phrased in the form of commitments. Inform all participants about the kinds of information they will be expected to bring.

You must answer the following questions (with these sample replies):

Annual Retreat Purpose? We would like our December meeting to have a very specific focus and that is on year-end review. It is very important that at the end of the year we re-evaluate our goals and set new goals for the new year.

Annual retreat content? What you will need for our meeting. Figure 5-9 is a sample of a retreat agenda.

Annual Review

Dear Doctor and Team: Please complete this before our meeting. Please consider all possible answers as potentially acceptable. We will brainstorm for the best and most feasible.

"We would like our _____ meeting to have a very specific focus and that is on conducting a year end review. It is very important that at the end of the year we re-evaluate our goals and set new goals for the new year."

You will need the following items for our meeting:
- A yearly calendar–staff and doctor report on any already scheduled seminars, vacations, holidays (federal and/or religious), team meeting schedules, etc.
- Our most recent profit and loss statement for a new calculation of the BEP and bonus incentive.
- Production and collection data to date for the calendar year in review.

Agenda

* Putting together a master schedule for _____ (year)
* Re-evaluation of goals
* Breakeven point review
* Vision re-evaluation and resetting (if necessary)
* Identification of barriers
* Brainstorming solutions to barriers
* Goal setting for _____ (year)
* Commitments for change for _____ (year)
* Copy of Mission Statement and Vision of the Practice to ratify.

* Ratify the Mission Statement and the Vision of the Practice. Do not move forward until both of these are improved and committed to paper.

I. List three accomplishments the practice has made in _____ (year).
   a. _____
   b. _____
   c. _____

II. List three accomplishments you have made in the practice in _____ (year).
   a. _____
   b. _____
   c. _____

III. Discussion of the goals for _____ (year); have we reached them?

Figure 5–9 Sample Agenda for an Annual Review/Retreat

IV. What would you like to see implemented in the practice in _____ (year)?

V. List three goals the team can work toward in _____ (year).

a. _____

b. _____

c. _____

VI. List three barriers that can keep the office from reaching these goals.

a. _____

b. _____

c. _____

VII. In order to reach our goal, we must identify our barriers, then develop possible solutions to these barriers.

List several solutions for each barrier that you believe will help solve this problem.

a. _____

b. _____

c. _____

d. _____

e. _____

f. _____

g. _____

VIII. Come up with three creative and polished suggestions and ideas to improve the following areas.

R	Laboratory	**0**	Inventory
1	Doctor's office	**2**	Physical space
3	Location	**4**	Front desk
5	Professional demeanor	**6**	Operatories
7	Team	**8**	Insurance
9	Marketing	**10**	Computer
11	Sales (case presentation)	**12**	Recall/perio
13	Scheduling	**14**	Morning huddles
15	Production	**16**	Staff meetings
17	Collection	**18**	Look at the office (try to put yourself in the patient's shoes and pretend this is a first visit)

Figure 5–9 continued

Communication Pearls: A Guide for Making Every Meeting a Success

New opinions are always suspected
and usually opposed without any
other reason but because they are not
already common. — John Locke

1. There are a number of "right" answers. Beware. Do not seek "the" answer.
2. You can contribute to a lot of "right" answers. Participate. Beware. Do not be shy.
3. Let others give their input. Listen. Build on what they say. Beware. Do not dismiss another's contribution.
4. Stay positive. Support your fellow participants. Beware. Do not criticize or scoff.
5. Look for quantity and variety. Beware. Do not dwell on any point too long.
6. Expand your thinking. Beware. Do not be constrained by conventional thought.
7. Address the subject, not personalities. Beware. Do not be exclusive with your ideas. Share them with the whole group.
8. Speak one at a time. Beware. Do not interrupt someone else's train of thought.
9. Stay loose and relaxed. Beware. Do not try to cover yourself.
10. Keep making suggestions. Beware. Do not give up.

Meetings succeed to the extent that communication succeeds. Please note that as you progress with these communication sessions over time, they will become special, and all team members will come to realize that the purpose of every meeting is to communicate and to excel. They are the team; they make up the practice. When they participate and focus on making the practice the best it can be, they will begin to autograph their work with excellence.

6 Knowing Your Patients

> *Knowledge itself is power.*
> — FRANCIS BACON

In chapter 5, we presented several agendas for meetings, emphasizing that every successful meeting has purpose and content. To reassess the importance of the hygiene department as it relates to the practice of dentistry, purpose and content must be examined in the context of how they relate to patient care. If we go back to basics, the *purpose* of every dental practice is to provide excellent care. The obvious corollary of this is that the *content* that is collected, shared, analyzed, and monitored in the practice must reflect this purpose. All must revolve around the patient. In short, it is the patient who provides the underlying agenda of every successful practice, and it is the patient who determines the professional and ethical agenda of the hygiene department. A true commitment to this philosophy begins with a thorough understanding of just who that patient is.

In general terms, the patient is the most important person in the practice—the only reason the practice exists. Thus, the patient should never be viewed as someone who interrupts the practice or as an inconvenience or an irritant. And while we are diligent in monitoring and analyzing practice statistics, we must always remember that patients are not just statistics. They are real people with real needs and real feelings. They bring their needs to us, and it is our responsibility to satisfy these needs and fulfill their expectations.

Patient expectations include dentistry that is skilled, reasonably priced, courteous, attentive, and up-to-date. In a good practice, every team member works to fulfill these expectations. In a master practice, every team member assists the hygiene department in providing dental care that exceeds these expectations. Knowing why things are the way they are helps.

THE DENTAL PATIENT AND THE SURGEON GENERAL

*A little neglect
may breed great mischief.*
— BENJAMIN FRANKLIN

In May 2000, the office of the United States Surgeon General released a comprehensive study on the status of oral health in America. It was, in many ways, a startling and uncomfortable indictment of the way things are and a call to action that has provoked much soul-searching in both the dental care community and the healthcare profession as a whole.

The nation's grade on oral health was a C-; the nation's grade on preventive dentistry was a C. Few states were above reproach, and far too many states failed in far too many of the areas under scrutiny.

Among the most important facts presented in the report was a confirmation that the mouth is indeed attached to the body. In and of itself, this is a simple fact that we all recognize. What is not as widely recognized is how neglecting what happens in the mouth can lead to or exacerbate serious illnesses not directly associated with the mouth. The Surgeon General's report not only corroborated the findings of previous independent research on this issue, it provided specific links between oral diseases and other illnesses and emphasized the importance of professional cooperation between dental health professionals and their medical colleagues.

The report confirmed that oral health problems could be symptoms of other health problems. It confirmed that oral health problems could cause or exacerbate cancer, diabetes, and kidney disease. It confirmed that undetected and untreated oral health problems could lead to bacterial infections that can seriously compromise many of the body's organs.

Statistics show that approximately 75% of the nation's adults suffer from some form of periodontal disease. The Surgeon General's report provides specific evidence that periodontal disease can be directly linked to low birth weight and premature births, to respiratory ailments and heart disease, blood clots, blood pressure fluctuation, and assorted other unhealthy and even life-threatening conditions.

The Surgeon General's report is a poignant reminder that preventive medicine is better than corrective medicine and that early detection is the key to early treatment, which can save not only teeth, but also lives. But while most practices have recognized the importance of preventive dentistry, few have made it a policy to provide a holistic approach to dentistry, which focuses not just on the mouth, but on the entire patient. This is not to imply that the dental health community has been negligent. But the time has come for *all* healthcare professionals, dental and medical, to make whole patient health a priority.

The Surgeon General's message is clear. Oral health as a significant component of overall health must be more seriously addressed in this country. The nation's policy on healthcare must be expanded to incorporate and implement meaningful and thorough attention to oral health. The report exhorts all healthcare professionals to monitor the oral health of their patients. It further identifies dental care professionals, and dental hygienists in particular, as those who are most able to perform this crucial task. Thus, it is the dental profession, and specifically the dental hygienist, who must take the lead in teaching policy makers and the American public that good oral health is critical to good general health.

The Patient, the Surgeon General, and the ADHA

It is ironic, but not entirely surprising, that the American Dental Hygiene Association (ADHA) recognized the connection between the body and the mouth at least five years before the Surgeon General's report. In the ADHA Code of Ethics for Dental Hygienists, which was approved and ratified in 1995, specific references to the correlation between oral health and total health are emphasized.

Under the Code's section on "Basic Beliefs," we find the following: "Dental hygiene care is an essential component of overall health care and we function interdependently with other health care providers."

Under the section on "Core Values," the ADHA further defines the hygienist's responsibilities: "Inform other health care professionals about the relationship between general health and oral health"

An even more telling item follows: "Promote a framework for professional education that develops dental hygiene competencies to *meet oral and overall health needs* of the public."

To live by this Code, we must improve our knowledge of the patients who are being served. It means knowing as much about those patients as we can. Some of this knowledge comes from general statistical information readily available to dental care professionals. The rest comes from individual patients. (Fig. 6-1)

Age-Related Dental Statistics

Carries Incidence

- 50% of children 5 to 17 years old experience cavities.

- 84% of 17 year olds have had at least one cavity.

- Root surface caries affect 20% of all employed adults and 63% of older Americans.

- By 64 years-of-age, 59% of all employed Americans (more than 50 million adults) have experienced tooth decay on at least one root surface.

Use of Sealants

- 11% of children aged 8 and 8% of adolescents aged 14 have received protective sealants on the occlusal surfaces of permanent molar teeth.

Incidence of Periodontal Disease

- 60% of adolescents age 15 have experienced gingival infection.

- After age 35, some form of periodontal disease affects roughly 3 out of 4 adults.

Figure 6–1 Learning about the Patient from the Statistics
Sources: National Institute of Dental Research: *Broadening the Scope: Long-range Research Plan for the Nineties,* 1990 (NIH Publication no. 90-1188); American Dental Association, *Survey of Dental Practices,* 1993.

Many dental practitioners have long been aware of the correlation between oral health and overall health. Few dental practices, however, have made the leap from awareness to action. Few have made the correlation a focal point of a proactive total health regimen for their patients. As we begin our comprehensive or periodic examination of each patient, the following age-related guidelines can be used during comprehensive evaluations (Fig. 6-2).

Remember, we are looking at our patients "from the tip of their heads to the bottom of their feet!"

Infant/Toddler (0-4)	Children (5-9)
Focus of Visit:	**Focus of Visit:**
Proper growth and development	Proper growth and development
Early intervention of care	Caries
Establishment of good attitudes toward care	Dentition development
Structural development	Gingival health
Eruption patterns	Interceptive orthodontics
Dietary issues/allergies	Maintain good attitudes towards health
Develop good oral hygiene skills	Develop good oral hygiene skills
Milk in bottle/nursing bottle caries	Language development
Language development	Neuromuscular development
Neuromuscular development	Structural delays
Developmental delays	Developmental delays
	Dietary issues/allergies
Preventive Education:	Medication/supplement usage
Baby bottle management	
Pacifiers	**Preventive Education:**
Oral hygiene education	Sealants
Caries education	Oral habits (sucking, bottle, fingers)
Antibiotic and supplement usage	Caries education
Occlusion	Antibiotic and supplement usage
Behavior development	Occlusion
Allergies	Behavior modification
Nutrition	Allergies
Primary vs. permanent dentition	Nutritional support
	Home care therapies
	Orthodontics and care of appliances
	Eruption patterns

Figure 6–2 Diagnosis and Education by Age

Adolescence (10-18)

Focus of Visit:
Growth and development
Orthodontic evaluation/maintenance
Gingival health
Nutrition
Mouth guards for sports
Caries
Medication interaction
Malnutrition/nutrition
Smoking/substance abuse
Dental health for a Lifetime
Self-confidence
Image

Preventive Education:
Pre-disposition to gingivitis
Nutrition
Medication interactions
Oral hygiene techniques
Orthodontics
Sealants
Mouth guard protection-traumatic injuries
Tobacco/smoking
Abused substances/effect on teeth
Oral cancer
Self-confidence

Young Adults (19-39)

Focus of Visit:
Healthy dentitions/keep teeth
for a lifetime
Medical/medicine Interactions
Gingival health
Caries reduction
Replacement therapy
Sports and/or mouth guards
Infant oral health care
Care during pregnancy
Nutritional counseling
Tobacco cessation
Lifestyle changes
Stress/depression/effect on dentition
Overall general health
Cosmetic dentistry

Preventive Education:
Oral hygiene instruction
3-, 4-, 5- or 6-months
  – Recare appropriate
Cosmetic dentistry
Care of crown and bridge
Sealants
Smoking
Oral cancer screening
Recession/root caries
Care of general health
Medication/supplement interaction
Stress reduction
Nutrition
Occlusion/grinding
Recurrent decay

Figure 6–2 continued

Middle (40-60)	Older (60+)
Focus of Visit:	**Focus of Visit:**
Overall general health-Surgeon	Balance between medical and dental health
General's report	Surgeon General's report
Medications/influence on oral health	Gingival health
Gingival health	Periodontal disease
Periodontal status	Lifestyle changes
Recurrent decay	Stress
Occlusion and grinding	Nutritional counseling
Nutritional counseling	Recurrent decay
Smoking cessation	Medication interaction
Lifestyle changes	Nutrition/eating habits
Cosmetic dentistry	Depression
Replacing missing teeth	
Depression	**Preventive Education:**
	Drug interactions
Preventive Education:	Xerostomia
Restorative/cosmetic education	Replacement of missing teeth
Periodontal awareness	Care of dentures/partials
Root caries/recession	Home care therapies
Medications/xerostomia	Systemic conditions and oral health
Nutritional counseling	Implants
Home care therapies	Prevention of root caries
Oral cancer screening	Recession
Systemic conditions and oral health	Nutrition
Surgeon General's report	

Figure 6–2 continued

Learning About the patient from the patient

Every practice has a new patient assessment form. The typical assessment form becomes a permanent fixture in the patient's file and includes general information such as name, address, telephone number, emergency contact, and the patient's version of past dental history. It generally includes at least cursory information about existing medical problems, the name and telephone number of a primary physician, and insurance information. During follow-up visits, patients in most offices are asked, "Have there been any changes in your medical history since your last appointment?"

This is not nearly enough. If we are to heed the recommendations of the Surgeon General and the ADHA and incorporate into our practices a holistic program that views oral health as an integral component of overall health, we need more. The "more" consists of two kinds of information: an assessment form that truly connects the body to the mouth and an assessment questionnaire that connects both of these to the patient's mind. The information is best collected during the initial comprehensive exam and then updated at least once a year. (Fig. 6-3)

Patient Name: _____
Appt: (New, Emergency, Recare) _____   **Date:** _____

Age: _____   **Height and Weight:** _____
Occupation: _____   **Years as a Patient in Practice:** _____
Personal History: _____   **Chief Complaint:** _____
Medical/Dental History/ Review of Systems/Medications/Supplements: _____

General Observations:

Physical:
Obvious physical impairments? _____
Use of special devices? (canes? walkers?) _____
At risk for physical emergency? (blood pressure, pulse, etc.) _____

Overall appearance:
Happy, depressed, secure, fearful? _____
Eyes - alert, bright, glassy, focused? _____
Dress and personal hygiene? _____

Substance Assessment:
Under influence of drugs? _____
Using medication? _____   Alcohol? _____

Emotional Assessment:
Eager to share or talk? _____   Dangerous to self? To dental team? _____
Emotionally stable? _____   Irritable? Frightened? Anxious? _____
Psychiatric problems? _____

Barriers:
Potential language barrier? _____   Potential cultural barrier? _____

Dietary/Nutritional Assessment: _____
Clinical Findings: _____
Extra and Intraoral Examination: _____   **Periodontal Examination:** _____
Dental Charting: _____   **Radiographic Evidence:** _____
Oral Hygiene Notes: _____
Dental hygiene treatment plan: _____

Figure 6–3 Dental Hygiene Patient Treatment / Assessment Form

Knowing the total patient means knowing the total patient

Some of the most important information you and your hygienist will need for a total and accurate assessment of the patient is information that can be gleaned only from examining the patient's frame of mind as it relates to dentistry, to your practice, and to the patient's perception of his or her own oral health and overall well-being. All too often, these attitudinal components are given minimal attention (or no attention at all). But if we are to treat the whole patient and not just an abscessed molar or a deep pocket in the left lower quadrant, we need to pay attention to where patients are emotionally and intellectually, not just physically. For this reason, every patient should be asked to supply a personal profile where these components are addressed:

PATIENT SELF-ASSESSMENT FORM

1. Why did you choose to come to our office at this time?
2. How do you feel about your past dental treatment?
3. What kind of image do you want to present to others?
4. How would you describe the general condition of your teeth?
5. If you could change the appearance of your teeth, what would you change?
6. How long have you been thinking of getting this treatment done?
7. What would it be worth to you to keep your teeth for the rest of your life?
8. If you had it to do over again, what would you do differently about your dental health?
9. How important is it to prevent future damage to these teeth?
10. How important is it for you to prevent expensive procedures sometime in the future?

The answers to these questions can be invaluable in determining treatment plans and procedures that are appropriate, acceptable, and feasible for patients. The responses should be incorporated into the patient's permanent chart and reviewed by the dentist and hygienist before any new treatment program is broached.

You should also consider compiling a Patient Introduction Sheet that provides general information about the patient's personal preferences, family, work, and other incidentals. (Fig. 6-4) Good communication is an essential part to holistic dentistry, and communication can be much enhanced by knowing something about the person you are communicating with.

---

1. Prefers to be called: _____

2. Family
    Single: _____
    Married: _____
    Children's names and ages: _____
    _____

3. Professional/Education
    Works for: _____
    Type of job: _____
    Attends: _____
    Year: _____

4. Social
    Feels strongly about: _____
    Personal information: _____

5. Relationship to practice
    Years in practice: _____
    New patient(s) referred:
    Name: _____
    Date: _____

Fig. 6–4 Patient Introduction Sheet

The Hygienist and Case Acceptance: Why Knowing the Patient Matters to Everyone

Always remember that knowing everything you can know about your patients is critical, and that the information gleaned from these preliminary assessments is worth its weight in gold. It is from this information that you build the groundwork for case presentation and case acceptance, the two components that keep patients coming back to your practice. Such patients are healthier and happier, and they help fulfill your practice productivity and profitability goals.

No one in the practice is in a better position to make this happen than your dental hygienist. The hygienist is the team member who can *build the relationship* that makes case presentation and case acceptance possible. She is the one who can best *share the practice philosophy* with the patient. She can *establish a need, instill knowledge and motivate,* and *ask for closure.* And in these elements lie the best-kept secrets of case acceptance.

Consider, for example, the potential power of the following hygiene scripts.

Philosophy Scripts

Mrs. Smith, our team has made a commitment to become the absolute best dental practice in town. As you can see from our brochure, our mission statement promises that we will help each and every one of our patients achieve the highest level of dental care possible. Did you know that the oral cavity is the "window" to the rest of the body? Many systemic conditions first manifest themselves in the oral cavity. This is why the doctor is committed to completing a very comprehensive exam on every patient.

You can keep your teeth for a lifetime, Mrs. Smith. Did you know this? I hope that after today's visit you will be eager to do what is necessary to maintain optimal dental health. Would you mind sharing with me the history of your dental health…Are you interested in the opportunity to keep your teeth for a lifetime?

Permission script

We will be completing a comprehensive exam and afterwards if you will let us, we will share with you everything we found during the exam. After we look at the results, we can decide together what you would like to do. Is this ok with you?

Establish the need and motivation script

To keep your gum disease from getting worse, we need to do a procedure called root planing. We can't do a regular cleaning because as you know from measuring the gums, they are very sensitive and we need to reach to the bottom of the pockets with our instruments. We numb your gums so when I use the special instruments, they will clean your root surfaces totally, so they are not rough and will become as smooth as glass. After we complete the procedure, we should get some healing and reattachment of the tissue to the tooth root. This will result in reduction of the pocket and lower pocket readings. How do you feel about making a commitment to a procedure like this?

Motivation script

Let me take a few moments to describe the benefits of having an implant placed in the area where you have lost a tooth. Is it all right with you if I share this information? An implant is the best opportunity for patients who have lost one or more teeth. It is like getting back your natural tooth. (Describe the features) We have seen hundreds of patients benefit from implants. I have (name a family member) with implants, and if I lost a tooth, I would immediately see if I could have an implant placed. Would you like doctor to see if this area would be a candidate for such a procedure?

Closure statements

I can bring the implant to Dr. Smith's attention if you would like me to.

Dr. Smith has outlined the treatment that he would like to complete. Do you have any questions about the therapy? I am happy to answer any questions you may have. Do you see yourself with this type of dentistry?

When Dr. Smith comes in for the exam he will decide which restoration will be best for that tooth. Here is a brochure about these two therapies, and I want to show you on this sample model exactly what we are talking about. You are looking at an investment of approximately $700-900. Do you have any questions about what I have just shared with you? Now I will get Dr. Smith to come in for the exam.

But potential is only potential until it is acted upon, and so we end this chapter on knowing your patients with a caveat. Knowledge in and of itself may be interesting, but without empowerment it remains dormant and virtually useless. For knowledge to truly become power, the person with knowledge must be empowered. In the following pages, we will present a case for this assertion, showing how empowering the *Pulse of the Practice* can make all the difference in the world.

7 Empowering the Pulse of the Practice

> Give me a firm spot on which to
> stand and I will move the earth.
> — ARCHIMEDES

THE COMPREHENSIVE EXAM: GIVING THE PULSE OF THE PRACTICE A FIRM SPOT TO STAND

No appropriate program of dental care can begin without a comprehensive examination. During this examination, the dental healthcare professional collects important information about the total patient: general physical health, health history, and oral health. The teeth and gums are checked thoroughly. X-rays are taken; images of potential problem areas are recorded by the intraoral camera. All problems and complaints are carefully noted.

In most master dental practices, the dentist completes the comprehensive exam while the hygienist performs all comprehensive recare exams on the "repeat, loyal customers." Regardless of the pathway the patient may take to the chair, in the master practice, the examination is the responsibility of the dental hygienist, who then reports her findings to the dentist. In either case, the practitioner has recognized and acknowledged that the dental hygienist should and must be involved in the comprehensive examination.

There are many reasons for this, the most obvious being that the dental hygienist is the staff member who spends the most time with patients, especially with patients who have come to the office for continuing care. By involving the dental hygienist from the start in the comprehensive exam, a dentist shows patients that the hygienist's participation and assistance are respected and important. Because patients see that the dental hygienist is valued by the dentist, their respect for the hygienist grows. Because they see the dentist entrust the hygienist with the important responsibility of performing the comprehensive examination, they are comfortable that they are in good hands. Because they respect and trust the hygienist, they are receptive to her advice and recommendations.

It is important to emphasize that patients' receptiveness to a hygienist's advice and recommendations for treatment is directly proportional to their perception of the level of responsibility given the hygienist by the dentist. The hygienist who is perceived as an active partner in the examination process is the hygienist who is perceived as trustworthy and capable. What patients trust, they esteem. What patients esteem, they listen to.

Most patients want to know what has been found during the comprehensive examination. They want to know about problems, solutions, and costs. Above all, they want the information presented in words that they can understand. The hygienist needs to keep all of these factors in mind.

"Let's review my findings before the doctor comes in to complete the exam. Tooth #3, your first molar, appears to have a fracture line right down the middle of the old silver restoration currently in the tooth. I believe that at this time it is best that we discuss with the doctor a more secure restoration for this tooth. The option would be a crown, or an onlay. Do you have any questions?"

The description is simple, clear, and specific. The hygienist has already established that corrective treatment will be necessary. She has also asked the patient to ask questions. Encouraging dialog gives the patient some measure of control over what comes next. The information presented to the patient should be restated and reinforced when the dentist comes into the operatory to complete the exam.

"Doctor Howe, I've shared with Mrs. Smith my concern about tooth #3. We know that the tooth would benefit from a more secure restoration. We've discussed the different options and I gave her brochures."

The hygienist's stature is further reinforced when the dentist confirms her findings and conclusions. Once a commitment has been made, the hygienist can introduce the patient to other team members who will participate in the process by scheduling follow-up appointments or by taking care of financial arrangements.

"Mrs. Smith, if you don't have any more questions, I'd like Susie to discuss the financial arrangements and schedule you for the onlay. Is this acceptable to you?"

"Susie, Mrs. Smith has made a commitment to have an onlay placed on tooth #3. Would you please assist her with scheduling the time and also work out the finances with her. I explained that the investment for the onlay is $850. She would like to utilize her insurance if she can, however, I told her that many insurance companies are not paying for the more permanent restorations, and that she may be responsible for paying for the procedure."

"Mrs. Smith, you have made a wonderful decision to have these permanent restorations placed. I have them in my own mouth and they are almost 20 years old now and just as perfect as the day they were placed. If you have any questions, or I can be of help to you, please do not hesitate to call me. See you soon."

By her active participation in the comprehensive examination, the dental hygienist has accomplished many things. She has introduced the patient to the practice and to individuals in that practice who will share the responsibility for the patient's overall well being. She has demonstrated her clinical skills and her knowledge of dentistry and dental procedures. She has encouraged the patient to agree to share responsibility for her own dental health and has motivated the patient to accept a positive solution to an existing dental condition. And through all of these steps, she has opened the door for a mutually beneficial lifetime partnership between the patient and the practice.

The PMV (Preventive Maintenance Visit) "It's not just a cleaning!"

Dental decay and gum disease afflict every man, woman, and child in the world. Neglected and untreated, oral health problems can become very serious, very painful, and very difficult to correct. Fortunately, modern dentistry in America makes it easy to catch these problems in their earliest stages, and dentists are able to control them before they become so debilitating and uncomfortable that they require expensive and extensive corrective procedures. The key lies in prevention.

As the fundamental building block of the recare program of the practice, the preventive maintenance visit (PMV) can no longer be viewed as "just a cleaning." It is a comprehensive session during which the master dental hygienist accomplishes two very important functions:

- Performing a wide range of clinical tasks and
- Providing information that will enable patients to make informed choices about treatment plans, services, products, and home care

In the hands of the master hygienist, a PMV will include the following:

1. A medical/dental comprehensive history update
2. Blood pressure/pulse screening
3. Oral cancer exam, extra/intra oral exam
4. Diagnostic x-rays (only the necessary ones taken)
5. Assessment of bone levels around the teeth
6. Plaque and tarter buildup assessment
7. Gum pocket measurements to determine the extent of periodontal disease
8. Check for tooth mobility
9. Complete oral exam
10. Sharing of the philosophy of practice
11. Wish list of the patient. Do you have one?
12. Exam of teeth for decay, cracks, broken and leaking fillings
13. Check of the gums for bleeding, inflammation, gum pockets, and breath test

14. Smile analysis and cosmetic dentistry evaluation
15. Tempro-mandibular Joint (TMJ) exam and bite analysis
16. Removal of deposits and stains above and below the gums— evaluation for periodontal therapy
17. Polishing with fluoride paste, air polishing with baking soda, and fluoride application
18. Personalized home care instructions and home care supplies
19. Review and update of individual dental treatment plans
20. Periodic examination
21. Irrigation with an anti-microbial solution
22. Tender loving care

The PMV requires knowledge, skill, integrity, and compassion. Patients should be fully informed about their condition, about the consequences of leaving the condition untreated, and about solutions and treatment plans. They should also be fully informed about time and costs associated with those treatment plans, and should be made to understand that the "twice a year checkup" may be upgraded to three or four times a year because it is not just a cleaning anymore.

TREATMENT EXPLANATION PEARLS: BE PREPARED!

- Think only in terms of optimum oral health
- Review what you saw on examination
- Help patient understand how each problem can be solved
- Explain why you chose specific treatment over alternatives
- Present only one treatment plan, the ideal one
- Explain probable prognosis if plan is not followed:
- "If we don't do this, here's what you can expect"
- Probe for any and all objections or concerns; address them
- Present total fee after treatment is understood
- Remember: explaining before treatment is a diagnosis…Explaining after therapy is an excuse

PATIENT EDUCATION: THE MOST IMPORTANT ASPECT OF PREVENTIVE DENTISTRY

It isn't that they can't see the solution. It is that they can't see the problem. — G. K. CHESTERTON

Too many dental patients do not understand how powerful preventive dentistry can be. Uninformed and under-educated, most do not value preventive dentistry. As dental professionals, it is our responsibility to teach patients what they need to know about the status of their teeth and gums to encourage preventive solutions before corrective solutions are needed.

Educating patients can be rewarding on many levels. As healthcare professionals, we want our patients to be healthy. A well-educated patient will be more interested in optimal dentistry than an ignorant patient. Education can make nervous patients less anxious. Knowing where they stand and knowing what can be done to improve that standing as comfortably as possible provide a powerful incentive to trust good dentistry. They will be less likely to miss appointments or cancel. Patients who are well educated are also easier to be with and to work with. Perhaps the most important benefit of patient education is the way in which it changes patient attitudes about visiting a dental practice. They stop being passive victims who are enduring terrible things in the dental operatory and become willing participants in improving their oral and overall health.

Teaching patients about oral health means knowing what you are supposed to teach. The educator, whether it is the dentist or the hygienist, should project expertise. This requires knowing everything there is to know about products, procedures, and technology related to maintaining healthy teeth and gums. Not knowing the answer to a patient's question may create the impression that your practice isn't as good as another practice. A lack of expertise diminishes the patient's belief in your ability and your skill. To prevent giving such an impression, your hygienist should project infallibility. She should read the professional journals, attend seminars, enroll in continuing education courses, and participate in professional study groups that focus on new research and technology.

Below is an extensive, but by no means total, list of dental therapies the master dental hygienist needs to know about:

- Whitening – both in office and at-home products
- Electric toothbrushes and other mechanical products
- Fluoride medicaments and programs
- Antibiotic therapy
- Periodontal rinses
- Micro-abrasion technique
- Lasers
- Occlusion
- Tooth-colored onlays/inlays
- Crowns
- Veneers
- Bridges
- Implants
- Composite restorations
- Sealants
- Night guards
- Occlusal splints/occlusal problems
- Endodontics
- Periodontal surgery
- TMJ therapy
- Oral surgery
- Extractions
- TMJ splints
- Orthodontic braces
- Periodontal surgery
- Injections, IV sedation, and oral sedation
- All post-operative treatment instructions
- Restorations—composites and gold
- Non-surgical periondontics
- Alternatives/supplements/nutrition
- Surgeon General's Report

She must also know how to communicate this knowledge to patients. If she is a skilled communicator, the dental hygienist establishes the needs and wants of the patients, and explains the best way to satisfy them. If her presentation is good, only minimal reinforcement from the dentist is needed to encourage the patient to accept the presented treatment plan. To be good, her presentation must be accurate. She must be certain that the facts she presents are precise and absolutely accurate. She must make the patient feel secure that he or she is in the hands of a competent professional who knows what she is talking about.

Good communication means being enthusiastic and assertive. The hygienist must always be aware of body language and tone of voice, because how we say something can impact credibility. She must believe in herself, believe in her dentistry, and consistently communicate to patients that the treatment she wants them to accept is the absolute best therapy for them. If the hygienist projects the slightest amount of doubt or hesitation, patients will "feel" it. To avoid this pitfall, she needs to learn the art of a confident and masterful delivery. This takes practice.

ALL THE WORLD'S A STAGE, SO WHY NOT TURN YOUR OPERATORY INTO A THEATER?

The dental hygiene department is the most important department in your practice. Your patients come here for their PMVs, for their cleanings, and for their periodontal problems. It is here that patients are examined for a variety of oral health problems and here that their overall physical health is routinely monitored. It is in the hygiene operatory that patients are educated about preventive dentistry, given instruction for home care, and taught about the value of routine maintenance. It is from your hygienist that they get initial information about a multitude of cosmetic and corrective procedures, ranging from porcelain crowns to devices that inhibit teeth-grinding while they sleep. And it is your hygienist who conveys to patients all the underlying information they need to begin a treatment plan or a rigorous maintenance program that is beneficial to their dental health and to the financial health of your practice. At least you hope so.

Unfortunately, the pretty scenario presented above is not always the case. While you hired your hygienist for her excellent academic credentials, her superlative clinical skills, and her enthusiastic and charming personality, these may not be enough. For while your hygienist may know everything there is to know about the subject of dentistry, she may not be communicating on this topic as well as she should be.

This should in no way imply that you have hired the wrong person for the job. It is simply a reminder that most good communicators aren't born—they practice till they get it right.

Consider stagecraft. No actor or actress worthy of the name appears on stage without preparation. They are given scripts. They are expected to memorize those scripts. And they are expected to rehearse and rehearse and rehearse until the lines they are to speak are letter perfect. And heaven forbid if those lines *sound* rehearsed! On the contrary, they must roll "trippingly off the tongue" and sound fresh and natural and exciting—even if they *have* been uttered twice a day for the last 28 days. Each matinee and each evening, a new audience comes to the theater. Every member of every audience expects to be transported to a different time and place through the power of words. A weak script can be enobled by a charismatic perform-ance. But even the best script will suffer if the performance is dull or wooden and sounds memorized.

So it is with dentistry. Information, no matter how critical or how interesting or how astounding, will not have much of an effect on your patients unless it is communicated in a manner that makes it worth listening to. And because there is more at stake here than a long running show or an extra encore, the communication skills of your hygienist are a thousand times more important than those of a Broadway performer.

Just as a brilliant actress plays to her audience, the effective hygienist must play to her patients. So what does this mean? The actress deals with an audience that, as a group, has essentially the same agenda. They have come to be entertained. The hygienist, on the other hand, deals with an entirely different audience. She may see five or 10 or 15 patients a day. None of these people are seeking entertainment. They do not sit in a polite group at a distance of at least 20 feet from her. "They" are an audience of one in a dental chair only a few inches away. Each one has an attitude, a concern, a problem, and at least one question.

In spite of the difference, the actress and the hygienist share one characteristic – both need to communicate in order to be effective at what they do. And both need to be students of human nature. An actress cannot portray a murderess, seductress, bag lady, or housewife without understanding something about people. A hygienist cannot communicate well to a bus driver or a teacher or even an actress without a full understanding that she is not just treating periodontal disease or a cavity or dry mouth. She is treating people who have needs and wants that far exceed the information they seem to be asking for.

Every day, your hygienist may be bombarded with dozens of questions from patients. The questions are asked from a perspective of fear, anxiety, skepticism, interest, denial, or even downright antagonism. For a hygienist to answer these questions effectively, knowledge of dentistry is only one of several essential ingredients needed.

A patient asks, "Why do I need x-rays? Are x-rays dangerous?" The question is actually two questions and reveals much about the patient's frame of mind and attitude. What we have here is a patient who is probably resistant to the idea of having x-rays taken *and* is looking for a way out. The hygienist has been challenged to give him or her a good reason to do so. The patient's tone may be whiny or annoyed. The patient may be concerned about cost or about unnecessary exposure to radiation. The hygienist who simply answers the questions at face value has not answered the questions at all. She has not responded to the annoyance or the anxiety or the financial concern that was the underlying reason for the question in the first place.

The first thing a hygienist needs to understand is that most questions patients ask do not pertain to factual knowledge. Most of these questions can be divided into five classifications: time, pain, finances, cosmetics, and value. Ironically, few patients ask about dental *health* unless it somehow pertains to one of these. Knowing that patients are motivated or inhibited by time, pain, finance, cosmetics, and value gives the hygienist a very definite advantage. It is the resource that allows her to answer all questions on two levels: informational and emotional. Once this has happened, she must have a script to match. Each script, of course, should combine dental fact with an empathy quotient that responds to a patient's emotional needs.

For example, the answer to "Why do I need a crown?" should present factual information about the purpose of the crown, which is delivered in a compassionate and understanding tone that recognizes and acknowledges the patient's anxiety about pain, time, and money. A skillfully delivered response will be listened to, not just heard. It will convey empathy, not just data.

A wonderful approach to optimal communication is to allow your practice to become a theater by giving your hygiene department time to create and rehearse scripts that achieve this fine balance between informational and emotional content. Scripts should be short enough to fit on a 3 X 5 index card and should be prepared on a variety of questions that patients are likely to ask:

1. Why do I need x-rays? Are x-rays dangerous?
2. Why can't I have a filling rather than a root canal?
3. Why can't you do this without anesthesia?
4. Why doesn't my insurance cover all this? They said it would at work.
5. Is this going to hurt?
6. What's the difference between a bridge and a partial?
7. What's the difference between a cap and a crown?
8. Aren't plaque and calculus the same thing?
9. How often should I change my toothbrush?
10. How often should I have my teeth cleaned?
11. Why do I need fluoride? I heard fluoride might be dangerous.
12. What are those sealants? Do they really work?
13. Why do you have to clean my teeth before doing the front tooth filling?
14. Why do I need to take pre-medication?
15. Can't I come in at 4:30? Or on Saturday? Do you have Saturday appointments?
16. Wouldn't it be less expensive to just pull my tooth?
17. My teeth have always been bad. Wouldn't dentures be easier/better?
18. Why are all of my new fillings sensitive?
19. Why do I have to see a specialist?
20. Why do I need a crown?
21. Can't you just put in another filling?
22. Aren't crowns expensive?
23. What's the difference between silver fillings and white fillings?

24. Gosh, that onlay sure is expensive, why does it cost so much?
25. How long will this onlay last?
26. Why can't you just fill my tooth instead of putting a crown on it?
27. Why are you here instead of the dentist?
28. I've never had a root canal. Everyone tells me they hurt. Do they?
29. I don't need to come in every three months to clean my teeth. They do not bother me. So why do you want me to come in so often?
30. I really do not have the money. What should I do now?

Encourage your hygienists to inject into their scripts an air of enthusiasm, humor, concern, drama, or even mystery as they answer these questions. Set aside some time for role playing and volunteer to participate by playing the patient. Make the project an in-service day and involve the entire dental team. Do not give up if everyone begins by being self-conscious. This is new and a little unnerving. It is likely that everyone will be hamming it up and making the scripts sound corny or melodramatic. In a short time, however, the stage fright and self-consciousness will wear off, and you may be pleasantly surprised at how well your hygienist can play the starring role in a variety of operatory scenarios. You will hear her provide information to a parent while settling an unruly child, soothe and comfort a dental phobic while explaining inlays, and charm the socks off the miserly grouch who thinks having all his teeth pulled is the optimal dentistry because it seems to be the cheapest.

Making the effort a practice project and involving the entire dental team show that you consider the exercise worthwhile. If approached enthusiastically and positively, it can motivate every member of the dental team to become better at communicating. The exercise will make your entire team better prepared to answer patients' questions. Rehearsing scripts will lead to increased self-confidence in responding to various situations and a variety of underlying emotional factors. It can lead to increased job satisfaction by reducing the exhausting and unrewarding frustration of giving a response and feeling that it has not been listened to. The role-playing can also help your team develop better listening skills as they learn to respond to cues thrown out by you, their coworkers, and their patients.

GENERAL RULES FOR CASE PRESENTATION

1. Always try to create a favorable impression of the practice.
2. Try to give patients what they want.
3. Always provide opportunities for patients to discover their own dental needs by asking questions.
4. Always raise the patient's expectations of what is possible. Share the "big picture."
5. Avoid presenting solutions to problems that a patient does not see as problems.
6. Never give the Dentistry 101 lecture to your patients. We are not here to lecture; we are here to educate. Know the difference.
7. Always ask questions that require a response from the patient. Never ask a closed ended question that requires only a yes or no answer.
8. Always explain treatment in terms the patient can understand and use visual aids whenever possible.
9. Always consider the patient's and your body language.
10. Always make direct eye contact. When presenting treatment you should sit knee to knee with the patient. Never stand above the patient.
11. Use permission questions and statements.
12. Always use closure statements.
13. Monitor the numbers related to case presentation or co-assessment.
14. Give patients a patient assessment form (Fig. 7-1).

PATIENT ASSESMENT FORM

During _____ 's appointment today we completed the following:

___Medical history update
___Oral cancer screening
___Periodontal screening
___Radiographs
___Periodontal therapy
___Antimicrobial therapy/irrigation
___Fluoride treatment
___Diagnostic study models
___Custom whitening trays
___Other evaluative procedures and/or referral

___Hard & soft tissue exam
___Cavity detection
___Oral hygiene instructions
___Dental prophylaxis
___Root planing, scaling
___Blood pressure/pulse
___Sealants, custom trays
___Whitening instructions

ORAL HYGIENE EVALUATION

___Good   *Very little plaque, calculus, stains*
___Satisfactory   *Some plaque, food debris, light bleeding, infection beginning*
___Needs improvement   *Plaque, calculus, stain present; tissue, inflamed & infected*

ORAL HYGIENE AIDS

___Toothbrush
___Super floss
___Toothpaste
___Interdental stimulator
___Other

___Antimicrobial rinse/Rx
___Threaders
___Fluorides/Rx
___Mouth rinse

___Floss
___Proxybrush
___Stimudents
___End tuft toothbrush

TREATMENT RECOMMENDATIONS

___Maintenance therapy at 3 months, 4 months, 6 months
___Daily home care maintenance with attention to
specific areas _____,
_____, _____
___Electric toothbrush - oral irrigator
___Sealants
___Radiographs
___Periodontal therapy intervention
___Dentistry recommendations:

_____
_____
_____
_____
_____
_____

Areas needing special attention

Upper Right Teeth   Upper Left Teeth

Bottom Right Teeth   Bottom Left Teeth

Figure 7–1 Patient Assessment Form

EDUCATING WITH THE INTRAORAL CAMERA

*Things seen are mightier than
things heard.*
— ALFRED LORD TENNYSON

For more than 10 years, dental experts have been extolling the virtues of the intraoral camera, designating it as one of the best tools available for educating patients about ideal dentistry. While many dentists still cautiously weigh the merits of this admittedly "pricey" equipment, those who have taken the leap soon recognize its benefits for their patients and for practice profitability.

The numbers have been calculated and the verdict is in. The first two new patients seen the first month the camera has been installed will cover the base payment on the camera. Consistent, proper utilization of the camera will increase case acceptance by as much as 30% per month. Those dental practitioners who subscribe to the theory that an educated patient is a patient who values optimal dentistry and accepts recommended procedures readily and consistently are not at all surprised by this correlation.

Once a dental practice makes the commitment to purchase an intraoral camera, the primary decision that needs to be made is about finding the best place to house the unit. Most practices decide to put the camera in the dentist's operatory. This is fine for the dental practice that has purchased a multi-operatory system. However, if the camera is utilized only by the dentist and only during new patient exams or treatment consultations, it is immediately devalued in this location.

In today's master dental practice, it is the dental hygienist who gathers the diagnostics, completes the preliminary exam, and predisposes the patient to the ideal treatment recommendations. The master dental hygienist co-assesses with the doctor, explains the treatment program, and puts closure to the treatment plan by asking patients if they "want" to commit to the therapy. Since the dental hygienist spends so much time educating patients, it is only natural that the camera becomes an integral part of the hygiene recare visit, especially when one considers that 40 to 80% of the dentist's scheduled therapy comes from the dental hygiene recare appointment. For all of these reasons, the ideal place for an intraoral camera is in the hygiene operatory with the dental hygienist.

While many hygienists are excited to have access to this wonderful educational tool, there is some concern about finding time to use the camera during the hygiene recare visit. Some hygienists worry about adhering to the tight schedules and about not interrupting the smooth patient flow that signals a busy and productive practice. To alleviate these concerns, establishing a time management protocol is advisable.

Good intraoral camera use begins with optimal timing. The patient and the hygienist review the patient's medical and dental history and discuss the patient's chief complaint. Radiographs are taken and momentarily set aside. Using the camera, the hygienist tours the patient's mouth. If time is at a premium, the tour can be curtailed and the hygienist can simply capture four camera images. While the patient is reviewing brochures on the dental procedure that is to be discussed or performed that day, the hygienist can excuse herself and go put the radiographs into the developer. Both the patient and the hygienist are engaged in performing some dentistry-related task throughout this interchange, and no time is wasted. The entire exercise should take about five minutes.

There are other pearls of wisdom that will help "camera shy" hygienists get started with the intraoral camera and utilize it to its best effect. Success with the camera is very dependent on attitude, and having a good attitude about the camera and its tremendous potential as the ultimate educational tool is especially important.

Purchasing the CD-ROM educational programs that are available with the intraoral camera is advisable. True proficiency comes with knowing all of the features of the technology. Trial and error learning can be costly, because some especially good features and capabilities of the technology may go undiscovered for years.

People who are especially successful with the camera begin using it the first day it arrives. Recognizing that a picture is worth a thousand words, they commit themselves to using the camera with every patient. Using this medium, a hygienist can initiate and nurture a relationship of mutual discovery. The patient sees with his own eyes what was previously only described in words.

Introducing the technology and the benefits to the patient can make the intraoral camera session much more effective. Give a demonstration of the camera's power by aiming the camera at the patient's ring, watch, or shirt. Using something the patient owns for the demonstration keeps the patient more involved in the process. As the camera magnifies the object it is focused on, say, "As you can see, Mrs. Smith the camera will magnify 20 to 30 times its original size, thus allowing both you and me a better opportunity to see your dental condition."

Positioning a patient for work with the intraoral camera is also important. The patient should be seated in an upright position. The camera should be down at the patient's foot or knee with the hygienist standing behind the patient so that both can see the screen. The camera should be glided gently through the mouth; the hygienist should comment on the images as they appear on the screen. This "live tour" of a patient's mouth is incredibly effective. As the lens moves through the mouth, and as the patient sees her teeth and gums on the screen, she becomes more involved and starts internalizing her dental condition.

The camera should be fulcrumed. Free-holding the camera out in the middle of nowhere will produce a blurry picture even with the steadiest hands.

Starting with the positive helps patients understand images of oral areas where there are problems. It is important that we show a healthy tooth first and then cross-reference with areas of concern. This prevents the patient from feeling overwhelmed or feeling that the hygienist is just looking for problems. Showing images of "better dentistry" is also recommended. The hygienist glides the camera around the arch until a normal, healthy, well-restored tooth is located. The ideal restoration can be used as a model for "better dentistry" that the patient may need at a later date.

Keeping it simple is critical. A hygienist who uses $50 dental words defeats the purpose. Communication happens only when what is being said is understood. Talking at the patient's level is not demeaning, it is merely common sense. "Look, this tooth is broken. It will require a more secure filling" and "See this black area? It's a very large, leaking, silver filling and it would benefit from a more secure restoration. Let's discuss your options, if you would like." are far more effective than any script that sounds like a description out of a scientific manual or textbook.

Involved patients are better patients. If the camera is equipped with remote control, the hygienist should let the patient have a turn at capturing an image. A patient involved in the process will retain more, learn more, and refer more. The camera photos will increase the "want," and this will reduce questions and objections to price.

Once the tour is completed and the patient has discovered personalized and visible dentistry, the hygienist should print two copies of the four-image photo—one for the patient's file and one for the patient to take home. After the financial presentation, the patient leaves the practice with a treatment plan, a brochure about the needed dentistry, and the photo. The visual impact remains long after the office visit ends.

Almost invariably, a dental practice that invests in one intraoral camera unit eventually moves to a multi-operatory system to accommodate each hygienist within the practice and the dentist as well. Not having to wheel the camera cart from room to room is the obvious advantage. The greater advantage becomes obvious to anyone using the camera even after a few weeks. By becoming experts in intraoral camera use, we raise our standards and we raise our patients' level of awareness. When these two complementary objectives are achieved, the way we practice dentistry is indeed enhanced.

CLOSING THE DEAL: GETTING PATIENTS TO REALLY WANT WHAT'S GOOD FOR THEM

One of the most fundamental truths about dentistry is that the most beneficial treatment procedure is useless if it doesn't happen. Too often, it doesn't happen because patients are taken only halfway up the road to optimal dentistry.

Making a treatment program happen is good for the patient and good for the practice and can be easier than you think. The magic formula that can turn a reluctant or unconvinced patient into a patient who is eager to accept the recommended treatment plan is effective education, *followed by an effective closing script.*

All people, including patients, want the best for themselves. This includes patients who resist treatment procedures. They resist because they do not recognize the value of the treatment the dentist or hygienist has recommended. They stop resisting when they truly understand that we are not just trying to sell them something, but are providing them with something that will protect, strengthen, and improve their oral health and overall health for an entire lifetime.

Properly educated patients know the exact nature of an existing problem, the short-term and long-term consequences of ignoring the problem, and the lifelong benefits of having the condition or problem treated; they will recognize that the procedures recommended by the dentist or hygienist are a cost effective and valuable investment. If your hygienist communicated these facts well, she has almost succeeded.

Almost is the operative word. All too often, this is where everything stops. The patient, thoroughly educated, is allowed to walk out the door and go home. The most important ingredient of the closing, getting the patient's commitment, has been omitted, and the best laid plans for getting the patient to come back for the recommended treatment procedures may have been unwittingly sabotaged. This is an especially unfortunate lapse, because it is at this point in the visit that getting a patient to commit to treatment is easiest. The groundwork has been laid, the patient has been well informed, the lessons on good oral health and good overall health are still fresh, and the concept of value has been communicated and understood. All systems are set to go, and the opportunity should never be ignored.

It is crucial at this point for the hygienist to follow through by asking for and getting a commitment. Asking "Can we go ahead and schedule an appointment to begin?" at this time will almost invariably get a positive response. Any residual resistance can be handled on the spot. Financial considerations, fear of discomfort, or anxiety about having to miss work to make dental appointments can be discussed and resolved as the molehills they are. If the patient goes home without making a commitment, these issues will most certainly turn into mountains and will be much harder to deal with.

Communication Pearls for the Dental Hygienist

The chief merit of language is clarity, and we know that nothing detracts so much from this as unfamiliar terms. — Galen

- Patients are not dental professionals. Effective communication begins with explaining things in language that they can understand.
- Patients who come to a dental practice are often anxious, sometimes in pain, and usually in need of compassionate and tender care. To communicate with patients effectively, the hygienist must present her information in a way that allows even the most terrified and uncomfortable patients to feel safe and sincerely cared for.
- No one likes bad news, and delivering a message about crumbling restorative work or receding gums is delivering news that is decidedly bad. Rather than accentuate the negative, a good hygienist will focus on solutions. It is wise to present the big picture by explaining to patients what benefits they will get from the treatment plans you propose and how these benefits will make them generally healthier. Explaining financial arrangements should be treated the same way. When giving the cost of a preventive procedure, for example, it is helpful to compare that amount with the amount that would be needed to correct an untreated condition.
- Whenever possible, involve the patient in the educational process. A very good way to do this is to use an intraoral camera. While you explain what you see, the patient is able to follow along—the information becomes much more real and your recommendations for treatment become more real as well.
- When educating new patients, enlist their cooperation by asking questions that will encourage them to ask questions about services and procedures available in the practice. Ask what kind of image they are interested in presenting. Ask what they would do if they

could change the appearance of their teeth. Ask how important it is for them to keep their teeth for a lifetime. Ask how important it is for them to prevent expensive procedures in the future. The power of suggestion is a vital educational tool and questions of this type make patients look beyond today's visit. They look ahead to optimal, lifelong oral health.

- Compliment patients who have made progress; encourage those who have not. Be specific, but do not condemn. Criticism makes people resistant. Education makes them understand the wisdom of doing things that will make them better.

- Last but not least, the dental hygienist should always remember that communication is a two-way street. She must always know when it is time to stop speaking and start listening. She must always be willing to give a patient her full attention. She must always be vigilant and notice when a patient signals through body language that he/she feels it is his/her turn to talk, to ask a question, to express an opinion, even to tell a joke. Only if this occurs is the circle of communication complete and unbroken. Only when this last condition has been fulfilled can the hygienist call herself a master communicator and educator. This can make all the difference in the world.

Figure 7-2 examines two ways to approach the issue of communication.

Scenario #1

Mary: Hi, John. Nice to see you. How are things?

John: Just peachy (grimacing). I've been having a really rotten day, starting with a really rotten dental appointment.

Mary: Sorry to hear that. What's up?

John: Well, to start off, my appointment, supposedly at 9:30, didn't happen till 10:15. These people seem to think I have nothing better to do than hang around waiting for someone to notice I'm there. Then they insist on taking x-rays even though they took them the last time I was there. Then they start poking and using that nasty mechanical thing to clean my teeth instead of the little pick. I complain that it hurts and nobody pays attention. I ask them to just use the little pick thing and they treat me like I'm a five-year-old having a tantrum. "Oh, Mr. Jones, it'll just be a few minutes and really, you can't tell me it hurts that much." Well, it did hurt, and I really didn't appreciate being told it's all in my head. I'm paying these people good money to take care of my teeth and I expect be treated like a person, not a body attached to a cavity. Then, to top it off, she starts telling me that I need an onlay or inlay or uplay or some such thing, and her explanation is so vague and weird I don't know what she's talking about until she tells me it's going to cost me seven hundred bucks. For that kind of money, I at least expected an appearance from the dentist himself—I guess he's out playing golf while the teeth pickers are running the business. On top of that, it's an investment that isn't going anywhere. Everybody's teeth fall out sooner or later, so why bother sinking money into all that fancy stuff? I think I want another opinion. Who's your dentist?

Scenario #2

Bill: Hi, Alice. Nice to see you. How are things?

Alice: Pretty good. I had a bit of an emergency this morning, but everything turned out better than I expected.

Bill: What kind of emergency?

Alice: I woke up with a really bad toothache and had to call my dentist to see if she could squeeze me in today. I had an appointment scheduled anyway for later in the week, but they agreed that it shouldn't wait, so they got me in pronto this morning.

Bill: Sounds like a great place.

Alice: They sure are. The people there are really good at what they do. My hygienist is especially terrific. Never keeps me waiting, always cheerful, always gentle. I always get the full low-down on what she's doing, why she's doing it, and how much it's going to cost me. If I'm not comfortable with something, all I have to do is make a face and she picks up on it and changes what she's doing or gives me an anesthetic. She really makes me feel like I'm a person, not just a bad tooth that happens to be attached to a body. Last month, when I had the flu, she even sent me a get well card! And the whole place is just as friendly and professional. I'm really happy with them.

Bill: Really sounds too good to be true. How long have you been going there?

Alice: For about ten years now and I'm planning to keep going back for as long as I have teeth. And according to my hygienist, I'm going to be able to keep my teeth for a very, very long time.

Bill: I haven't been to a dentist in years—never could stand the—but I really think I should start going again. Yours sounds like a winner. Do they take new patients? Do you happen to have their phone number?

Figure 7–2 The Dental Hygienist: A Patient's View

In the two case scenarios presented, one dental practice lost a patient and another dental practice kept a satisfied patient and is about to gain another through a referral made during a chance encounter and casual conversation. Both events occurred through the simple process we call "cause and effect." The effect is easy to spot. John is leaving his dental practice. Alice is holding onto hers for dear life. Bill, who hasn't been to a dentist's office in years, is about to make an appointment with Alice's dentist. And Mary, after hearing John's story, will probably think her dental practice isn't so bad after all.

In each case, the cause is almost as easy to read as the effect. On the surface, the patients seem to be responding to the practice in general. Dig a little deeper, and you will find that in each case the most important factor under consideration is the hypothetical patient's view of the dental hygienist. To John, the hygienist is a "tooth picker" who doesn't deliver much besides physical and financial discomfort. This colors his perception of the entire practice. He is obviously unhappy with the care he is getting, with the cost of treatment, and with what he perceives as indifference to his dental health and indifference to him as a person. Alice, on the other hand, sees her dental hygienist as a caring, pleasant, dedicated professional who is working with her patient to ensure a lifetime of good dental health. Her glowing description of the practice begins and ends with the hygienist. Her hygienist is not just a "tooth picker"—she is a partner in the fight against cavities, gum disease, pain, and tooth loss. It is her praise for her dental hygienist that has made Bill reassess his attitudes about the dental profession. We know that Bill is going to call to make an appointment at Alice's practice, just as we know that nothing in the world would induce Mary to check out John's dental practice.

Let's look at some of the specifics. National statistics tell us that between 40–80% of dental care needs are found during the 50 to 60 minute dental hygiene appointment. During those 50 to 60 minutes, the hygienist may update a patient's medical records, perform fluoride therapy, take x-rays, perform prophylaxis, or perform innumerable other tasks. As the member of the dental team who provides the treatment that helps prevent oral disease, she performs some of the most important functions within a dental practice.

Statistics also show that up to 95% of all dental patients have some level of gum disease. Here again, the hygienist's services are indispensable. As a well-trained professional, she collects and reviews data, performs comprehensive examinations of hard and soft tissue, and discusses with the dentist and with the patient appropriate treatment and follow-up care for both the dental office and home.

These are awesome responsibilities that require excellent clinical skills and a thorough knowledge of dental products and procedures. But even the best product cannot be sold without appropriate packaging and marketing. The hygienist is often the one who makes patients decide to come back or stay away.

As the person in the practice with whom patients have the most contact, the hygienist must be the practice's best goodwill ambassador. This begins with effective time management. Just as no dental hygienist should cool her heels in the operatory because of a no-show, no scheduled patient should have to that cool his or her heels in the waiting room. Permitting this to happen makes patients like John feel they are not being treated with respect. Respect breeds respect; it is mutual. John feels he is not being treated with respect, that he is "body attached to a cavity." He returns the favor tenfold by referring to his hygienist as a "tooth picker." Alice, who feels she is treated with respect, has no problem expressing how much she respects her dental hygienist and, by extension, the dental practice that is smart enough to employ such a gem.

Respect goes hand in hand with overall attitude. One of things valued by patient Alice is "caring." The hygienist has taken steps to show Alice that she matters, not just as a dental patient, but also as a person. During their sessions, she is cheerful. Because mood is contagious, this matters. When Alice was home with the flu, the hygienist sent a get well card. While this is not an earth-shattering event, it is just the kind of small gesture that makes another human being feel good. From John's tirade, we get the feeling that his hygienist would never have thought of making such a gesture.

Every interaction with a patient is going to be a positive or negative experience that affects patient loyalty, retention, and referrals. Since most patients in a dental practice spend most of their time with the hygienist, it is she who bears the heaviest burden of providing customer service that is positive and attractive. This means selling herself and presenting herself in the most positive way she can. Alice's dental hygienist has done this very effectively. Her patient views her as a competent and skilled professional who provides excellent care. John's hygienist falls far short of the mark. He complains that she is not gentle, does not listen well, and doesn't acknowledge his need to feel comfortable. She has violated three of the cardinal rules that every dental hygienist should live by: to be gentle, reassuring, and perfectly tuned in to a patient's needs. She has made no effort to make her patient feel important.

Alice and her hygienist have a relationship that is based on mutual respect and a mutual commitment to Alice's good dental health. Because her hygienist's goal is to make certain Alice keeps her teeth for a lifetime, Alice believes this can happen and feels a real connection to her hygienist and the practice. John, on the other hand, has no personal connection to his hygienist. She is, in his view, an underling that is taking care of things while the dentist is out golfing. In John's eyes she is just the hired help, and she has apparently done very little to change his mind. Unlike Alice, John believes that tooth loss is inevitable, a good reason not to bother with regular maintenance and restorative treatments. His hygienist has not been an effective educator.

It is the hygienist's responsibility, more than anyone else's, to make patients aware of their dental problems and to explain the consequences of those problems if they are not treated. Clearly Alice's hygienist has succeeded in conveying these important ideas to her patient. Alice believes. She does not complain about money; it is obvious that she feels comfortable investing in her smile and in her good dental health. It is just as clear that John's hygienist has missed a golden opportunity. When John grumbles about "onlays or inlays or uplays" we get the impression that he really missed something. His hygienist didn't bother to make sure he understood the treatment procedure and the need for it. The only thing that registered with John was the cost. Because the hygienist did not take the time and the care to instill in John a belief in the value of routine maintenance and restorative procedures, he views both as a bad investment.

Every professional providing a service to clients, customers, or patients should know the value of self-promotion. Dental hygienists are no exception. Every day brings new challenges and new opportunities to make patients view you as a professional who has the ability, the skill, and the competence to make their lives better, healthier, and more comfortable.

Ignore the opportunity and "John" will be a regular in your practice—that is until the day he decides to leave. If your hygienist does her job and rises to the challenge, all of your patients may turn into "Alice"—happy that she has found her dental wonderland, content to stay there, and more than willing to let others in on the fun.

8 The Dental Hygiene Periodontal Program of Care

> Nothing can be created out of
> nothing. – LUCRETIUS

In the preceding chapters, we have emphasized that the core of a thriving master dental practice is a thriving hygiene department. For this concept to be truly workable, it must be based on the premise that a hygiene department thrives to the extent that its central focus is a well-developed periodontal program of care.

PERIODONTAL THERAPY —AN OVERVIEW

There are four basic phases to periodontal therapy. Any practitioner, whether a general dentist, a hygienist, or a periodontist, needs to pay attention to these four phases.

The first phase is plaque control

This is basic and important to any form of dental therapy, whether it is periodontal or restorative. The patient's health and dental history play a major role in the *direction* of the therapy.

A prophylaxis is an attempt to remove those factors that facilitate the progression of periodontal disease. This is done by removing plaque and calculus from tooth surfaces and is generally limited to deposits at the gingival line. A simple prophylaxis is usually a one-visit procedure.

The second phase is tissue control

This phase involves the management of both hard and soft tissues so that infection can be controlled. In this phase, the tissue is treated by scaling and root planing, or by surgical therapy.

Scaling and root planing refer to the treatment of root surfaces that lie within periodontal pocket spaces. The instrumentation, as well as the approach, is different than for simple prophylaxis. The aim of the clinician is simply to clean and polish the teeth in the prophylaxis. Scaling and root planing are ways of treating pathologically deepened pockets and contaminated root surfaces.

The third phase is occlusal analysis and control

A patient's occlusion may or may not relate to his periodontal disease. If, after careful assessment, occlusal factors are found to be related to a patient's periodontal disease, they must be treated.

The fourth phase is the maintenance phase

This phase entails the patient and the therapist working together to control the treated case. Notice that all of the phases involve control. It is important to realize that periodontal disease has to be *controlled.* It is not cured by performing certain treatments.

When we get into the maintenance phase, some of the research shows that plaque control is not necessarily as important as the frequency of recare to remove toxins. We can do a lot to maintain our patients after they have been treated. We don't have to take the attitude that a patient who practices less than ideal hygiene is a "bad guy."

The bad side of this is that we tend to take it personally when patient cooperation is lost. The motivation of patients to perform good home care is an ongoing process that involves a close, cooperative effort between the therapist and her patients.

THE PERIODONTAL PROGRAM GONE MISSING: HOW TO BRING IT HOME

The dental profession claims that 90–95% of dental patients have some level of gum disease. If this is so, then why does the average dental practice maintain fewer than 15% of its dental patients in some level of a periodontal program? In some cases, a comprehensive periodontal program was never incorporated into the practice. In other cases, a program was instituted and then abandoned. The lament I most frequently hear is, "Well, we *had* a great periodontal program! We don't seem to be into it as we were once before!" "Our patients don't really care about coming back every three months!"

In a master practice, neither scenario is acceptable. In fact, every master practice should be achieving, at a minimum, a 98% case acceptance rate for conservative periodontal therapy. This holds true for practices that never had a periodontal program to begin with and for those practices where a periodontal program existed and died from neglect.

Integrating or resurrecting a comprehensive periodontal program into your practice takes the same time, dedication, and energy as restructuring your practice to enhance and augment your hygiene department. Each team member plays a key role in the overall success of the program. Every person on the team must work cohesively to convince patients that new treatment approaches will help them. In other words, the team will have to rethink old values, establish goals, and learn all aspects of the therapy, which will require exquisite verbal skills and a proactive attitude. Once you make the commitment, there can be no turning back.

Before objectives can be clear, the team must think about its purpose. Each team member must make a paradigm shift and put new philosophies into practice. This includes defining specific objectives, and the most important of these are related to your managerial skills.

PERIODONTAL PROGRAM OF CARE OBJECTIVES FOR THE DOCTOR

As you move forward with the clinical/managerial growth of your practice, you will need to ask yourself some important questions. Some of them will be difficult, and some of the answers will be even more difficult, because they will indicate a need for more changes and additional adjustments that need to be made within the entire practice.

The most basic question of all is whether everyone in the practice knows what periodontal disease is and how gravely periodontal disease can affect both oral health and total health. If not, education in varying degree and detail is essential.

Your first responsibility will be to teach everyone in the practice to begin thinking "outside the box." The most important lesson will center on treatment of a whole patient. Everything else, including the manner in which your periodontal program develops, will stem from this.

Job duties will need to be reviewed, revised, and redirected to accommodate the program. All should be committed to paper.

Decisions will need to be made about the entire process of patient evaluation. Who will see the patient during the first visit—the dentist, the hygienist, or both? Who will collect periodontal data? How often is periodontal data collected? Is the data collection process dramatically different for new patients and recare patients?

Upgrading and standardizing periodontal charting is essential. Is the periodontal charting you currently use adequate? What is the ratio of periodontal screenings to full mouth probing with recorded numbers? Is there a protocol on how often a full mouth probe should be done? Are the forms you currently use good enough? Do they need to be revised, refined, or scrapped and replaced? Does periodontal charting routinely go hand in hand with a comprehensive review of every patient's medical history? If different team members are involved in charting, are charting and documentation consistent?

You must also carefully review classification protocol. This begins with a critical look at periodontal literature and documentation your team has access to. Is the practice using the most recent AAP Periodontal Classification? Is each patient being properly and systematically classified into the appropriate level of health and periodontal disease?

When disease is noted, does the hygienist spring into action by presenting the patient with treatment plans and therapies? Is patient education about periodontitis standard operating procedure in every operatory? Is current literature on all stages of gingivitis and periodontitis available for distribution to patients? Are all team members committed to continuing education that will allow them to participate in the patient education process?

Has a cost analysis of the hygiene department's periodontal program been done? How much does it cost to run? What would it take to make you comfortable with the profitability level? Have you considered differentiating fees for periodontal screenings and examination procedures? Have you developed a specific fee protocol for long-term periodontal therapies? For periodontal maintenance? Have you considered what you and your hygienist need to do to re-educate patients who visit a dental practice twice a year and have a condition that warrants three or even four annual visits?

There are additional questions and issues that must be addressed with the entire team. All of them echo the pattern that makes hygiene the pulse of practice; all of them are indispensable units in the creation of a rock-solid periodontal program of care.

There must be a written periodontal philosophy firmly in place, and every staff member must be aware of this philosophy and fully supportive of it. The practice vision must be reflected in the periodontal philosophy, and the periodontal philosophy must be an extension of the practice vision. Both should be "living" concepts whose principles are made "real" on a daily basis. They should be words to live by, not words to frame and mount on a wall and seen out of the corner of the eye.

All team members, not just the hygienist, must learn to be effective communicators. All must learn how to deal effectively with barriers put up by patients who resist optimal periodontal care. Continuing education in clinical management is a must. Continuing education for your hygienist and the rest of the team, at seminars, accredited institutions, or in-house, is just as important.

Treatment planning should be systematic and patient specific, not generalized and haphazard. Many variables, including behavior modification and nutritional analysis, must be considered before any treatment plan is designed and recommended to any periodontal patient.

Home therapy programs must be evolved just as systematically and must be everyone's responsibility. Consistency must be maintained throughout.

Your version of optimal home therapy cannot be at odds with the version of the hygienist in Operatory 1. The hygienist in Operatory 2 and the dental assistant and front desk team member must present patients with home-care philosophy and protocol that are substantially similar in content, execution, and implementation. The infantry, the cavalry, and the commander-in-chief need to march to the same drum-beat, for it is only in this manner that the practice presents each patient with a united front that is firmly committed to a single cause.

Among the most important issues you must address is your own ability to think "outside the box" by keeping an open mind that is capable of perceiving possibilities in new products, techniques, and technologies. Many of these can truly bring your practice periodontal program to the cutting edge of new millennium dentistry.

PERIODONTAL DISEASE AND THE DENTAL HYGIENIST

The dental hygienist plays one of the most important roles in implementing a comprehensive periodontal program. The hygienist is responsible for collecting thorough data on each patient. The exam includes, but is not limited to, reviewing the chief complaint, taking the necessary radiographs, completing a comprehensive soft tissue exam, and noting hard tissue changes.

After the diagnostics are obtained, it becomes the hygienist's responsibility to educate and stress the importance of ideal dental health. The verbiage utilized by the hygienist must be direct, yet compassionate in delivery. The following script can be utilized during the examination.

"I am going to complete a periodontal exam. I will gently probe around each of your teeth and check the tissues. I will be using a small rounded instrument with millimeter markings on it from 1-10. It is called a periodontal probe. I will be measuring the level of bone. (Describe how periodontal disease progresses.) I will call off several numbers. When I call out 1-2-3, these are considered normal readings, but anything above 1-2-3, such as, 4-5-6-7-8-9-10, means there is a gum

pocket or a gum swelling; a concern with your gingival tissue.
If I find anything like that, I will go over it with you when we
are done measuring. Is this acceptable to you?"

This is merely the tip of the proverbial iceberg. The work of the hygienist as the core of the practice periodontal program is far more complex and has a much greater impact than most dental professionals realize. To understand the full significance of the hygienist's role in periodontics, it is crucial to examine the objectives that are germane to a successful, productive, and profitable periodontal program.

PERIODONTAL PROGRAM OF CARE OBJECTIVES FOR THE HYGIENIST

As the team member who will be most involved in presenting and implementing periodontal therapy, your hygienist will need to work with every patient and every other team member. She must help educate the entire dental team about the etiology of periodontitis and about non-surgical approaches to periodontal treatment. She must motivate other team members to become excellent patient educators and must set a sterling example for others to follow by improving and refining her own communication skills, both verbal and non-verbal. Above all, she must set an example of positive and proactive professionalism.

The fact that your hygienist should have excellent clinical skills is a given; the fact she should be equally skilled in diagnostic principles is not as widely recognized. A hygienist who has graduated from an accredited institution, has maintained a professional interest in her specialty, and has committed herself to improving her knowledge and skills through continuing education is formidable. She knows, for example, the connection between periodontal disease and certain medications, stress and anxiety, puberty, smoking, poor nutrition, genetics, pregnancy, bruxism, and other systemic diseases. She also knows what to look for and knows, as well, that what she finds in the oral cavity is assuredly interrelated with an entire person. Thus, granted the autonomy that is her due and is in the best interest of the practice, it is the hygienist who should set guidelines for periodontal therapy, beginning with total patient assessment.

It is the hygienist who should evaluate the periodontal status of each new patient, using the latest classification provided by the American Academy of Periodontology. It is the hygienist who should chart periodontal findings, using the most comprehensive form available or a form she herself has designed for optimal efficiency and custom-made accuracy. (A cautionary note on this is that the practice cannot function well if every hygienist has custom-designed charting paraphernalia. In practices with more than one hygienist, custom-designed charts should be a team project reviewed by the practitioner).

Once a thorough assessment of a patient has been made and properly documented, it is the hygienist who should present to that patient a detailed and individualized treatment plan. The plan should stipulate precisely the following points:

- What the initial treatment will entail
- What recare and maintenance protocol must be adhered to
- What home-care activities the patient will need to take responsibility for
- What the treatment will cost
- What the patient risks by not accepting the treatment plan
- What costs are involved in accepting or not accepting the plan
- What short-term and long-term benefits the patient will derive from the recommended treatment

It is the hygienist who should re-evaluate and monitor all continuing care patients and the hygienist who should lead the campaign to convert every patient's old oral health habits and patterns to more effective, appropriate, and individualized regimens.

While it is best for each patient to work with the same hygienist during each stage of the treatment plan, scheduling considerations and other variables may make this impossible. In practices with more than one hygienist, continuity and consistency are critical. The flow of therapy, like documentation and assessment formulae, should be standardized. Thus, one of the most useful tools for hygienists is a comprehensive (non-periodontal) form where general information, medical information, treatment plan information, and attitudinal information can be recorded. While general in scope, Figure 8-1 shows how compiling seemingly unrelated information about a patient provides an in depth profile that can be of assistance to any member of the team that deals with the patient.

Patient Name _____ **Date** ___/___/___

Hygienist: _____ **Chief Complaint:** _____

Expected Treatment for the day:

Recare _____ months

Evaluation _____ months

Fine scale _____

SC/RP _____ now _____ later

Oral irrigation _____

Perio referral _____ now _____ later

Antibiotic therapy _____

Other _____

Discussed with Patient:

New recare interval _____ Evaluate in near future _____

Fine scale _____ SC/RP _____

Antibiotic therapy _____ Periodontal treatment _____

Restorations needed _____ Other: _____

Inlays _____ Crowns_____ Bridges_____ Implants_____

Full/Part denture _____ Composites _____ Whitening _____ Veneers_____

Night guard _____ I.V. sedative _____ Onlays _____ Sealants_____

Other _____

Patients Reception/Attitude of Proposed Treatment:

Asked for commitment? _____ yes _____ no Outcome? _____

Negative _____

Disbelieving _____

Probable acceptance _____

Will/may need reinforcement from Dr. _____

Full acceptance _____ Financial concerns _____

Other _____

Figure 8–1 Dental Hygiene Communication Form

Every hygienist should be apprised of every patient's insurance coverage as it pertains to periodontal coverage. Often, knowing what is covered and what is not is a crucial component in case presentation. Knowing how to assist the patient in maximizing the insurance coverage for periodontal therapy is also critical. It is often the deciding factor that encourages a reticent patient to commit to treatment.

In the operatory, the hygienist should handle with equal dexterity all clinical facets of periodontal therapy as well as all peripheral facets that contribute to a patient's well being. This includes providing nutritional information that relates to periodontal tissue management, reviewing and explaining radiographs with patients, and discussing products that will assist the patient in better home care.

Each hygienist should also be actively involved in scheduling and marketing, two areas that will be discussed in greater detail in subsequent chapters.

THE COMPREHENSIVE PERIODONTAL PROGRAM: THE FIRST KEY TO SUCCESS

Individualized treatment planning is the key. After the appropriate documentation is collected, a diagnosis is made, and the patient is presented a treatment plan that can be implemented. When preparing the periodontal program, use the following criteria for diagnosis of periodontal disease:

Periodontal Classifications

(Some of the definitions of class types are currently pending an upgrade by the Academy of Periodontology)

Class 0   Health
Tissue   Healthy pink color, stippled, no inflammation or bleeding
Pockets   0-3mm; no bone loss; no mobility
Deposits   Light plaque and no calculus

Class I   Gingivitis
Tissue   Inflamed; bleeds 20-30 seconds after probing; sensitive to touch; presence of bleeding and/or exudate; changes in gingival form.
Pockets   Not more than 3–4 mm; no bone loss or mobility.
Deposits   Light scattered deposits of calculus (requires little time to remove)

Class II   Early (Slight) Periodontitis
Tissue   Inflammation into deeper periodontal structures; a fine line of blood when probed.
Pockets   3–4 mm with slight loss of connective tissue attachment; slight horizontal bone loss (possibly); no mobility.
Deposits   Generalized sub-gingival; deposits are harder to remove.

Periodontal Classifications continued . . .

Class III   Moderate Periodontitis

Tissue   Recession; anterior teeth drifting; inter-dental triangle fills with blood; heavier bleeding.

Pockets   5–6 mm; noticeable loss of bone support and increased mobility; angular and horizontal bone loss on x-rays.

Deposits   Generalized tenacious moderate to severe sub-gingival deposits and infection deep into pockets.

Class IV   Advanced Periodontitis

Tissue   Fibrotic and bulbous; red; bleeds very easily and profusely.

Pockets   7+ mm; major loss of alveolar bone support usually accompanied by increased tooth mobility; sever recession; sensitive to heat and cold; posterior furcations; mobility 3+.

Deposits   Deep, tenacious deposits with exudate, plaque, and debris.

Class V   Refractory Periodontitis

Characterized either by rapid bone and attachment loss or slow but continuous bone and attachment loss. There is resistance to normal therapy and the condition is usually associated with gingival inflammation and continued pocket formation.

Further Classifications

A. Early Onset Periodontitis
- Pre-Pubertal Periodontitis
- Localized
- Generalized
- Generalized
- Juvenile Periodontitis
- Localized

B. Periodontal Disease Associated with Systemic disease

C. Acute Necrotizing Ulcerative Gingivitis

ASSESSING THE TOTAL PATIENT

Assessing the "total patient" additionally requires us to look at some risk factors that may be present that will affect the outcome of our therapy and, ultimately, could affect the overall health of our patients. These risk factors include, but are not limited to the following:

- Health history – Family history, age, gender, diet, weight, level of activity, smoking, high blood pressure, lifestyle
- Current drugs and their interaction – xerostomia, halitosis
- Genetics – Diabetes, HIV, leukemia, osteoporosis

- Dental considerations – Loss of teeth, implants, mouth-breathing, overhangs, frenum pulls
- Current health behaviors – Tobacco use, alcoholism, age (menopause), stress diet/nutrition, drugs

Once the patient is classified, the appropriate treatment forms are presented. The following is a sample of what the treatment plan form could look like for a patient diagnosed as a Case Type II:

Class II – Early Periodontitis	
First Appointment	**Second Appointment**
Periodontal root planing	Periodontal root planing
Periodontal root planing	Periodontal root planing
Irrigation, per quadrant	Irrigation, per quadrant
Irrigation, per quadrant	Irrigation, per quadrant
Home fluoride	Electric toothbrush/other
O.H.I	O.H.I.
Third Appointment	**Case fee for the total** _____
Fine scale & polish	4- to 6-week - re-evaluation appt.
Periodontal probing	Recare – 3 or 4 Months
Irrigation, per quadrant	Other – Agents for application
Irrigation, per quadrant	Other – Services to be presented
O.H.I.	

Figure 8–2 Early Periodontitis

As the patient reviews the written treatment plan (Fig. 8-2), the hygienist continues with the verbal presentation of the periodontal condition and the recommended therapy. Remember, "It's not what you say, but how you say it." Developing strong verbal skills can mean the difference between patient acceptance of periodontal therapy and refusal of treatment. A script, which can explain the benefits of the root planing procedure, follows:

"Your present periodontal condition is classified as chronic periodontitis. This means that your tooth-supporting structures are starting to weaken. Your gums show signs of pocket formation. The treatment will require very thorough cleanings of the gum, including root planing, which will

smooth the tooth surface and remove the toxins deep inside the pocket, so the tissue can reattach. If you would like us to, we can numb your gums, so you can remain comfortable. After we complete the procedure, we will closely monitor your success. The key word I use to explain monitoring is control. We want to control the disease, because science has not yet discovered a total cure for well-established periodontal disease. For this reason, once the treatment begins, it will be emphatically important for you to continue your home care efforts and come here to the office to see me for your maintenance visits, every three months. Do you have any questions or concerns about what I have shared with you? Tell me how you feel about making a commitment to these therapies."

It is important to ask patients if they are absolutely clear on the recommendations and put closure to the case by asking if the therapy presented that day is what they want to have done. If patients really want the dentistry, they will show up for appointments.

Remember, explaining before treatment is a diagnosis; explaining after treatment is an excuse!

Treatment Plan Objectives

- Halt disease progression and stabilize periodontal attachment levels
- Repair periodontal tissue
- Maintain oral health

Treatment Protocol

- Initial assessment
- Periodontal exam (probing and radiographs)
- Presentation of patient treatment plan
- Risk factor assessment (smoking, diabetes, family history)
- Patient commitment
- Therapy

Treatment Plans

Non-Surgical Therapy
- Scaling and root planing
- Patient education
- Home products
- Scaling or root debridement
- Irrigation

4-6 Week Re-evaluation
- Retreat areas
- OHI
- Product referral (antibiotics, irrigants, other, etc.)
- Full mouth re-probe
- Prophylaxis

3 Month Supportive Periodontal Therapy
- Update medical/dental history
- Oral hygiene assessment
- Evaluating patient's emotional/cognitive response to therapy
- Patient education and home care review
- Periodontal maintenance
- Clinical and periodontal exam
- Evaluating patient's physical response to therapy
- Risk factor review
- Supra-gingival, sub-gingival scaling and/or root planing

Surgical referral if necessary

Figure 8–3 Steps to the Dental Hygienist's Successful Perio Treatment

FORMS FOR PATIENTS

The old maxim, "put it in writing," is nowhere better applied than in the practice of dentistry. This is especially the case when presenting patients with a comprehensive multi-phased treatment program. Because we all risk dealing with patients who accept a treatment program only to turn around and back out of a program in mid-stride, some versions of Figures 8-3 through 8-9 are indispensable. Consider printing your forms so that they will tear-off with a copy for the file and the original to the patient.

A firm, yet flexible radiographic protocol must also be determined for your practice (Figs. 8-3 thru 8-11)

(Gum inflammation, Attached connective tissue involvement, slight bone loss on x-rays, 3–4 mm probing depths)

First appointment – approximately 1½ hours

Comprehensive exam
Periodontal probing w/exam
Irrigation
Oral hygiene instruction
Home products introduced _____

Full mouth X-rays
Debridement before diagnosis
Fluoride treatment for sensitivity
Home aids introduced _____

Second appointment (UR/LR) and Third appointment (UL/LL) – approx. 1½ hour each, optimally in one week

Oral hygiene review and reinforcement
Quadrant scaling and root planing with anesthesia
Quadrant scaling and root planing with anesthesia
Full mouth ultrasonic irrigation

Fourth appointment (approximately 1 hour, optimally one week)

Oral hygiene review and reinforcement
Fine scaling
Fluoride treatment for desensitizing
and anti-cariogenic purposes

Full mouth ultrasonic irrigation
Polishing
Recare – Three (3) months

Other recommendations:

❏ Soft bristle brush	N/C	❏ Sonicare	$
❏ Floss (w or w/o threaders)	N/C	❏ Braun	$
❏ Inter-proximal brush	N/C	❏ Hydrofloss	$
❏ End tufted brush	N/C	❏ Rotadent	$
❏ WaterPik	$	❏ Toothpaste	$
❏ Chlorhexidine rinse	$	❏ Mouth rinse	$
❏ Antibiotic Therapy	$	❏ Other	$
		Total: _____	

I request and authorize the doctor and/or such qualified assignees to perform the dental work listed above.

Patient Signature _____ **Date** _____

Figure 8–4 Early Periodontitis (Class II)

(Gum inflammation, Attached connective tissue loss, Moderate Bone loss on x-rays, 4–6 mm probing depths)

First appointment – approximately 1½ hours

Comprehensive exam

Periodontal probing w/exam

Irrigation with chlorhexidine

Oral hygiene Instruction

Full mouth x-rays

Debridement before diagnosis

Fluoride treatment for sensitivity

Second, Third, Fourth and Fifth appointments
Approx. 1 hour each, optimally in one week

Oral hygiene review and reinforcement

Full mouth ultrasonic irrigation with chlorhexidine

Quadrant scaling and root planing with anesthesia

Sixth appointment (approximately 1 hour, optimally one week)

Oral hygiene review and reinforcement

Full mouth ultrasonic irrigation with chlorhexidine

Fine scaling

Polishing

Fluoride treatment for desensitizing and anti-cariogenic purposes

Other products _____

Other recommendations:

❑ Soft bristle brush	N/C	❑ Sonicare	$
❑ Floss (w or w/o threaders)	N/C	❑ Braun	$
❑ Inter-proximal brush	N/C	❑ Hydrofloss	$
❑ End tufted brush	N/C	❑ Rotadent	$
❑ WaterPik	$	❑ Toothpaste	$
❑ Chlorhexidine rinse	$	❑ Mouth rinse	$
Recare – 3 months		❑ Other	$
		Total: _____	

I request and authorize the doctor and/or such qualified assignees to perform the dental work listed above.

Patient Signature _____ **Date** _____

Figure 8–5 Moderate Periodontitis (Class III)

Appointment 1:	Fee
Comprehensive exam	
Periodic exam	
Intraoral-complete series (including BW)	
Panorex film	
Bitewings – 2 Films	
Bitewings – 4 Films	
Intraoral – Periapical first film	
Intraoral – Periapical additional film	
Intraoral – Periapical additional film	
Intraoral – Periapical additional film	
Prophylaxis – Adult	
Prophylaxis – Child	
Topical application of fluoride - Adult	
Topical application of fluoride - Child	
Oral hygiene instruction	
Home products	
Case Fee	

Figure 8–6 Case Type: Controlled (Health)

Appointment 1:	**Fee**
Periodic exam	
Comprehensive oral exam	
Intraoral – complete series (including BW)	
Panorex	
Bitewings – 2 Films	
Bitewings – 4 Films	
Intraoral – periapical first film	
Intraoral – Periapical additional film	
Intraoral – Periapical additional film	
Intraoral – Periapical additional film	
Intraoral – Periapical additional film	
Full mouth debridement	
Palliative treatment	
Oral hygiene instructions	
Appointment 2:	
Prophylaxis adult	
Adult fluoride	
Oral hygiene instruction	
Products to take home	
Case Fee	

Figure 8–7 Case Type: Gingivitis

Appointment 1:	**Fee**
Periodic exam	_____
Comprehensive oral exam	_____
Intraoral complete series (including bitewings)	_____
Full mouth debridement	_____

Appointment 2:	**Fee**
Periodontal scaling & root planing per quad	_____
Other _____	
Periodontal scaling & root planing per quad	_____
Other _____	
Oral hygiene instructions	_____

Appointment 3:	**Fee**
Periodontal scaling & root planing per quad	_____
Other _____	
Periodontal scaling & root planing per quad	_____
Other _____	
Oral hygiene instructions	_____
Recommended home products	_____

Appointment 4:	**Fee**
Prophylaxis	_____
Oral hygiene instructions	_____
Adult fluoride	_____
Home products recommended	_____

Recare 3-Month	**Fee**
Periodontal maintenance	_____

Case Fee	_____

Figure 8–8 Case Type II – Slight (Early) Periodontitis

Appointment 1:	**Fee**
Initial oral exam	_____
Periodic exam	_____
Comprehensive oral evaluation	_____
Intraoral complete series	_____
Full mouth debridement	_____
OHI, home products reviewed	_____

Appointment 2:	**Fee**
Periodontal scaling & root planing per quad	_____
Periodontal scaling & root planing per quad	_____
Application of desensitizing medicaments	_____
OHI, home products reviewed	_____

Appointment 3:	**Fee**
Periodontal scaling & root planing per quad	_____
Periodontal scaling & root planing per quad	_____
Application of desensitizing medicaments	_____
OHI, home products reviewed	_____

Appointment 4:	**Fee**
Prophylaxis (fine scale/polish)	_____
Periodontal re-evaluation	_____
Oral hygiene instructions	_____
Adult fluoride	_____

Recare Appointment: (3-Month Intervals)	**Fee**
Periodontal maintenance	_____
Oral hygiene instructions	_____
Adult fluoride	_____
Home products reviewed	_____

Case Fee	_____

Figure 8–9 Case Type III – Moderate Periodontitis

Appointment 1:   Fee

Initial oral exam
Periodic exam
Comprehensive oral exam
Intraoral complete series
OHI, review of home products

Appointment 2:   Fee

Periodontal scaling & root planing per quad
Periodontal scaling & root planing per quad
Oral hygiene instructions
Application of desensitizing medicaments
Subgingival irrigation

Appointment 3:   Fee

Periodontal scaling & root planing per quad
Periodontal scaling & root planing per quad
Oral hygiene instructions
Application of desensitizing medicaments
Subgingival irrigation

Appointment 4:   Fee

Fine scale, Re-evaluation, polish
Periodontal probing
Oral hygiene instructions
Adult fluoride
Subgingival irrigation

Recare Appointment: (3-Month Intervals)   Fee

Periodontal maintenance
(Does not include the exam)
Oral hygiene instructions
Adult fluoride
Review of home products

Case Fee

Figure 8–10 Case Type IV – Advanced Periodontitis

The following radiographs will be taken on Patient X _____	
Intraoral – complete series (including bitewings) Frequency:	$ _____
Panoramic film Frequency:	$ _____
Bitewings – two films Frequency:	$ _____
Bitewings – four films Frequency:	$ _____
Intraoral periapical – first film Frequency:	$ _____
Introral periapical – each additional film Frequency:	$ _____

Fig. 8–11 Radiographic Policy

It is important to understand that these forms are not just extraneous paperwork.

Each of them provides patients with information that assists them in making educated decisions on periodontal care recommended by the hygienist. Each of them has a major impact on whether or not patients accept treatment in the first place and then stick with the program with a total commitment to optimal oral and total health.

They are the building blocks of getting your patients to understand, accept, and comply with optimal periodontal care.

PATIENT COMPLIANCE

The patient must combat the
disease along with the physician.
— HIPPOCRATES

A broadly accepted definition of the term "compliance" is "the extent to which a person's behavior coincides with medical and health advice." When dentists were questioned about what patient behaviors concerned them most, non-compliance with oral hygiene instruction ranked high. In the periodontal office, many of our best therapeutic efforts are doomed because of non-compliant behavior.

Studies show that only 51% of patients given oral hygiene instruction were in the "high compliance" group; 38% were classified as "moderately compliant," and 11% were "non-compliant," within 30 days after oral hygiene instruction. Non-compliance manifests itself in two specific modes:

- Failure to return to the dental practice for recommended treatment programs and
- Failure to practice good home care

Studies show that most patients do not brush optimally, much less use suggested inter-proximal aids. Another study reported that a significant number of patients drop out of recommended oral hygiene regimens. Two-thirds of the patients who drop out of such treatment programs do so within 90 days.

WHY PATIENTS FAIL TO COMPLY

I would prefer not to.
— HERMAN MELVILLE

Denial

In some cases, non-compliance is a manifestation of denial. Patients simply choose not to believe the serious nature of their dental illness. Many tend to be highly dependent and want someone else to take care of them. In their view, the therapy for their illness is someone else's responsibility. Home care is neglected entirely or practiced sporadically and inefficiently because the underlying premise is that the problem should be taken care of at the office. The reasoning is that they are paying to have someone else deal with the problem and should not have to be bothered dealing with it themselves.

Patients who "can't be bothered" are patients who are unmotivated or uneducated. Successful communication techniques can work wonders in improving compliance in this group. The dentist or hygienist (or both) needs to explain fully and thoroughly any existing problems, any and all consequences of leaving the problem untreated, consequences of neglecting home care, and benefits to be had from regular office visits and efficient home care. This information needs to be presented in simple layman's terms that can be easily understood. A confused patient is not an informed patient and will find it easy to slip back into denial and non-compliance. Make sure any questions or uncertainties are addressed and handled. Encourage patients to call to discuss any residual questions or concerns that may occur to them after leaving the office. Keep the home care drill simple. The simpler the required behavior, the more likely it is to be carried out. Put what you say in writing.

Provide positive reinforcement. Most people do better with positive feedback and resist negativity and criticism. Remember that patients are people too and avoid the temptation of criticizing—taking a negative approach can give patients a new excuse to slip into the same non-compliant pattern.

Fear

Fear is a major factor of non-compliance in dentistry. Fear often prevents patients from visiting a dental office at all. It is one of the primary reasons patients break appointments and abandon a recommended hygiene treatment program altogether.

Modern dentistry has made most dental procedures painless and comfortable. If a patient is fearful or anxious, that patient is either uninformed or is reacting to previous painful and uncomfortable dentistry. In some cases, changing the behaviors of dentists and hygienists toward patients is advisable. Many dental care providers tend to think of "good" patients as those who are not anxious where dentistry is concerned. Anxious and fearful patients tend to be viewed as "bad" patients. Their fears and anxieties are often perceived as irrational; dealing with them takes time and energy. Providing assurance (and reassurance) is the best antidote. This should never be condescending or vague. Trivializing a patient's fear will get you nowhere; vague claims like "this won't hurt a bit" are useless because they do not explain why the treatment or procedure is painless.

For extreme dental phobics, other approaches are advisable. These can include group education or videotaped motivational/educational programs for fear reduction. Changing the entire dental team's attitude to use a system of positive reinforcement should also help to improve compliance and alleviate fear.

Money

Economic issues also lead to non-compliance, especially for patients who believe fixing a dental problem is a one-visit proposition. Many of these patients believe that everything that ails them can be and should be handled in the dental office during a single visit. The prospect of paying for long-term maintenance that keeps a dental condition in check and prevents further deterioration is viewed as an unnecessary expense. There are also those patients who truly cannot afford the fees for long-range periodontal programs without financial assistance. In many cases, these patients have no idea that financial assistance is available from a variety of sources.

Help from third-party payments has been one way of reducing the problem. In lower socioeconomic groups, monetary rewards have been shown to improve compliance. Patients who can pay but won't pay are a different matter altogether. These are patients who have not been properly educated to recognize that preventive dentistry and a maintenance program are more cost effective and valuable than expensive corrective procedures that are inevitable if prevention and maintenance are not practiced. A few simple mathematical home truths, which point out the difference in dollar amounts for prevention and dollar amounts for corrective procedures, can be very enlightening to such patients and can improve their attitude about compliance quite effectively.

Patient dissatisfaction

In a recent study, 60% of the patients queried cited the dental team's indifference (or perceived indifference) as the main reason for non-compliance and/or leaving a dental practice altogether. The average dental practice experiences a 50% patient turnover every five years. A full 50% of this turnover is attributed to patient dissatisfaction. At this time, there is no concrete evidence that all of these patients move on to other practices. It is generally assumed that many simply drop out and subsequently seek out dental services only when a condition becomes so painful or uncomfortable it is impossible to ignore.

This self-destructive behavior is most often a direct result of poor customer service. Patients expect good, prompt service. They also expect to be treated compassionately and to have their concerns and their problems taken seriously and addressed with respect. If these conditions are not met, they walk. The more your practice and your suggestions fit patients' needs, the more likely they are to comply. Satisfied patients tend to do more of the recommended home therapy than dissatisfied patients. Satisfied patients also tend to come back for recare appointments. Assume responsibility for ensuring that this happens.

Failed appointments create problems for both the patient and the office. Reminding patients of appointments is acceptable and appropriate. Many will appreciate the extra attention. Keep records of compliance. Patients can "get lost in the system," and every effort should be made to make sure they are found and brought back to the fold. This may require diligent maintenance of computerized record keeping systems or a more hands-on approach of routine chart reviews to relocate and reactivate patients who have disappeared without a trace. Without the patient, there can be no patient compliance.

IMPROVING COMPLIANCE

Simplify, simplify.
— HENRY DAVID THOREAU

Simplify. Patients tend to remember what you tell them first. The simpler the required behavior, the more likely it is to be carried out.

Accommodate. The more your practice and your suggestions fit patients' needs, the more likely they are to comply. Satisfied patients tend to do more of the recommended therapy than dissatisfied patients.

Remind patients of appointments. Failed appointments create problems for both the patient and the office. Patients break appointments for various reasons. Communication is a key element, along with a perceived need for the visit.

Keep records of compliance. Patients can "get lost in the system" and efforts should be made to keep up with them. This may require advanced systems, possibly the use of a computer.

Inform. Put what you say in writing and give a copy to the patient. This and other exercises of the dentist's authority have been recommended as ways to reduce non-compliance.

Provide positive reinforcement. Most patients do better when positive feedback is given when compared with a more negative approach to their compliance problem.

Identify potential non-compliant patients. If there is suspicion that compliance will be absent or erratic, discuss the problems that this may create for the patient before therapy begins.

Remember that in medicine and dentistry, compliance tends to be poor in patients who have chronic diseases they perceive as non-threatening.

COMMUNICATING THE VALUE OF FLUORIDE

Patients treated by dental hygienists tend to fall into two categories: periodontal healthy and periodontal unhealthy. For periodontal healthy individuals, the treatment objective is simple—disease prevention. When a periodontal problem exists, we tend to recommend therapies that will prevent the establishment of periodontal pathogens within plaque. One of the most widely utilized products available to us is fluoride.

When discussing fluoride treatments with patients during a hygiene appointment, it is very important to stress the benefit of the product. We know that incorporating fluoride into home or office treatment plans has many benefits. Fluoride kills pathogenic bacteria in plaque. It prevents or slows the re-colonization of periodontal pathogens in plaque and oral tissues.

We also know that many patients refuse fluoride treatment because it represents an out-of-pocket expense. Fluoride treatments are preventive, and in spite of the current emphasis on the benefits of preventive medicine, they are one of a host of preventive procedures that too many insurance companies categorize as beyond "usual and customary." When patients learn that payment for a fluoride treatment will be their responsibility, they find a reason to resist the treatment.

Dealing with patients who refuse to accept a recommended treatment plan and complain about the cost of a recommended plan means understanding the true reason for the resistance. In most cases, the problem is not financial, but educational. Somewhere along the line, the value of the treatment procedure has not been effectively conveyed.

This is a problem that should be addressed quickly and thoroughly. Patients who are well-informed will stop resisting when they truly understand that their dental practitioner is not just trying to sell them something, but is providing them with something that will strengthen, protect, and improve their oral health for an entire lifetime.

Effective communication involves the use of excellent authoritative sources. Citing the recent Surgeon General's report on how oral health problems can cause or exacerbate general health problems and relating this information to the preventive benefits of fluoride can often bring about the desired compliance. Citing preventive guidelines established by the American Dental Association can be equally effective. This is especially true when dealing with the parents of pediatric patients, especially when those patients are among the 40 million American children who live in areas of the country where water supplies are not fluoridated. It is important to share with these parents, in particular, specific ADA recommendations for fluoride:

Age 6 months to 3 years	*.25 mg daily*
Age 3 years to 6 years	*.5 mg daily*
Age 6 years to 16 years	*1.0 mg daily*

In children, fluoride is primarily important as a caries deterrent. In adults, it reduces plaque volume, inhibits new caries, and decreases sensitivity. For adults, the ADA recommends preventive in-office fluoride treatments and prescription fluoride gels and pastes for home use to supplement in-office treatments.

Reinforcing an oral presentation on fluoride with visual aids is crucial. Patients can be given brochures, copies of research articles, or written materials prepared by the office staff. Questions should be encouraged and answered simply, accurately, and convincingly. All costs should be specified up front. They should be presented not as an expense, but as an investment in oral health. If this information is delivered correctly, it is not only educational, but also motivating, and few patients will fail to make a commitment if one is asked for at this time.

It is important not to underestimate the power of timing. Given enough time to "think things over," even a thoroughly educated patient can manage to convince himself he can get by without it. For this reason, it is advisable to get a commitment to the treatment while the patient is still in the chair.

SAMPLE PATIENT LETTER

Our office has re-evaluated our fluoride recommendations. We now recommend the application of fluoride gel following routine dental cleanings for children and adults. Fluoride can safely prevent decay, reduce sensitivity, and is beneficial in the treatment of periodontal (gum) disease.

Fluoride can be administered in two basic ways. Using prescribed fluoride tablets strengthens un-erupted developing teeth. Teeth that have already erupted benefit from topical fluoride in various forms. Our goal is to provide optimal dental care for our patients. The use of fluoride is an important aspect of keeping your teeth at their best.

ADA Recommendations for Fluoride

Age — 6 months to 3 years	*dosage - .25 mg daily*
Age — 3 years to 6 years	*dosage - .5 mg daily*
Age — 6 years to 16 years	*dosage - 1.0 mg daily*

For adults, the recommended fluoride treatment therapy will provide the following benefits:

- Desensitization
- Retards recurrent decay
- Kills disease causing bacteria

We recommend a treatment at each preventive appointment and also a prescription for fluoride gel to use at home. The hygienist will recommend the brand and type best for you.

A Dozen Pearls for Developing an Excellent Hygiene Periodontal Protocol

1. Hold departmental meetings once a month. Doctor must be present. Hygiene coordinator runs meeting. Rotate scheduling of departmental meeting to fit the schedule(s) of hygienist(s). Make sure minutes are provided to all members of the team (See Chapter 5 for sample agendas)

2. Utilize the following diagnosis/evaluation tools when creating periodontal protocol:
   - Probe readings – six points documented once a year
   - Bleeding index – Gingival index Grade 0-3
   - Radiographic guidelines
   - Medical/personal/dental history
   - Comprehensive examination

3. Have hygiene update necessary radiographs. Protocol is to update the full mouth radiographs every 3-5 years. Consider seven vertical bitewings once a year (if necessary). When updating bitewings, consider four verticals as well.

4. Create a customized treatment plan based on diagnosis/evaluation.

5. Hygiene presents periodontal recommendations to patient after history, blood pressure, radiographs, probing, OHI education, and all other needed diagnostics are completed. Utilize AAP case types 1-5.

6. Once diagnosis is confirmed, present the need for advanced dental hygiene care using the word crossroads. "Mrs. Smith, we have come to the *crossroads* with regard to your periodontal health. You have to make a choice."

7. Prepare the operatory to handle the presentation and present the image you want to project. Utilize numerous visual aids to help you in treatment planning and presentation of therapy. Find and adopt good forms, documents, brochures, and other helpful aids that can help the patient grasp the level of disease and what action must be taken to arrest the condition. Practice scripts.

8. After the treatment plan is presented and before you touch a scaler to a tooth, close the case and get a commitment to treatment. Make sure to give patient a copy of periodontal charts. Once the patient says yes, begin customized treatment therapy.

9. Review with patient the technology and equipment to be used:
   - Root planing instruments
   - Intraoral camera
   - Computer
   - Probing system

10. Other recommended products for home care:
    - Oral irrigators
    - Electric toothbrushes
    - Mouth rinses
    - Toothpastes
    - Antibiotic therapy
    - Oral hygiene aids

11. After therapy is completed, schedule appointment for reevaluation (4-6 weeks)

12. Patient is scheduled every three months for periodontal maintenance.

9 Recare, Retention, and the Pulse of the Practice

All is number. — PYTHAGORAS

Recare is defined as patients returning to a dental practice for continuing care appointments at least twice a year. Recare is not to be confused with simple recall cleanings. It is a never-ending process of educating your patients about periodontal disease and proper oral hygiene. Because recare involves education and reinforcement from the moment a patient enters the office, it is critical that every person in the practice realizes the role he or she plays in this ongoing process.

A properly run recare department will contribute 30–45% of the annual gross production of a practice. Even more telling is the fact that 40 to 80% of the annual gross production of a doctor's treatment comes from hygiene recare chairs. For this reason alone, your hygiene recare rate should be 85% or better. One hundred percent of the patients seen by the dental hygienist should make appointments for continuing care. Up to 75% of patients should and can be referred to a more frequent recare schedule. Up to 50% should be referred to a more intensive level of periodontal treatment. Less than 10% of your patients should be lost through cancellation or broken appointments.

Evaluating how your hygiene department's statistics compare to these percentages is critical. The numbers you come up with determine your productivity; your rate of productivity determines your profit. If your dental hygiene department's statistics don't measure up, decide to make them measure up by setting numerical goals. Monitor numbers daily, weekly, monthly, and annually. Analyze the data you collect and learn from them. These data can be your most important tool for reading patterns and trends. They can also help you spot warning signs early enough to deal with problems effectively, appropriately, and proactively.

The success of your recare program can be measured by one vital statistic: how many patients come back for treatment on a regular basis as frequently as you or your hygienist recommend. To determine your success rate, you need just three numbers:

- The number of active patients in the practice,
- The average number of recare visits each month, and
- The average number of months between recare appointments you prescribe.

For example, if your practice has 2000 active patients and the average recare interval is 5.5 months, you should have no fewer than 290 recare appointments per month. Thus,

$$290 \times 5.5 \div 2000 = 80\%$$

Rating the Health of Your Recare Department

Super	80% or better
Excellent	70-80%
Good	60-70%
Fair	50-60%
Poor	below 50%

How does your practice compare?

Determining Hygiene Recare Efficiency

Facts are better than dreams.
—Winston Churchill

The American Dental Association (ADA) reports state that the average dental practice has a 50% or less recare effectiveness annually. Monitoring recare efficiency enables you to judge how your practice stands. It can provide the foundation for keeping those patients as repeat, loyal customers. Using the following computations will help you assess recare efficiency:

- Count the number of patients due for the current month.
- During this month, count the number of patients that actually complete their recare appointment for the designated month.
  Example:
  A patient was put on a 6-month recare and was due in December 2001. If the patient was seen 12/18/01, the visit would be counted as a recare. If the patient was seen 1/3/02, the visit would not be counted as a recare, simply as a hygiene appointment.

- Number of patients that complete recare appointments **X 100 =** recare efficiency
  Example:
  If **250 =** patients that completed their recare appointments, and **310 =** patients that were due for recare that month, then:
  250 ÷ 310 = 0.81 X 100 = 81% recare efficiency
  Thus, 19% of the recare patients for that month were not seen.

The Pre-Appointment Recare System

The most efficient recare system to use is the "Pre-Appoint System." Its advantages are threefold:

- It allows the office to attain an 85% or greater recare efficiency
- It implies a commitment from the patient for regular dental care
- It guarantees continued growth in the hygiene department

The most effective way to implement this system is as follows:

1. The hygiene book appointment schedule or computer screen should be listed in 10-minute intervals just like the doctor's. This will allow for a more efficient scheduling of time than the usual 45-minute time frame allotted to hygiene in most dental practices. (Who would know better the time required than the person who just completed a treatment)?

2. Each patient receives an appointment for the appropriate return date from his or her current appointment date.

3. The appointment should be made in the hygiene operatory by the hygienist while she is waiting for x-rays to develop or waiting for the doctor to examine the patient.

4. The patient self-addresses a postcard that will be mailed as reminder of the appointment. The card will have the appointment day, date, and time on it. You may also want to include the length of time that will be required for that appointment. Make sure the postcard used is bright and eye-catching.

5. The card is then filed in a file box subdivided into months and weeks. For example, cards are divided as January 1-7, January 7-14, January 15-21, January 22-31, etc. This box may be kept at the front desk or in the hygiene operatory.

6. The appointment card is mailed no earlier than two or two-and-a-half weeks prior to the appointment. This allows the patient enough time to call and confirm or change the appointment. Please check each card before mailing for any time or date changes.

7. A confirmation call should be made two days prior to the appointment. This will allow enough time for the office to fill any changes that may occur in the schedule.
8. The confirmation is a front desk duty; the objective of the hygienist is to work herself back into the operatory and produce dentistry.
9. An interval recare card should always be kept alphabetically by the month the patient is due.

NINE WAYS TO INCREASE HYGIENE RECARE APPOINTMENTS

1. Two days before the scheduled appointment, phone the patient and reconfirm the time and date. Mention, again, the purpose of the recare and the time that will be required for the appointment. If you have difficulty contacting patients during the daytime, try to contact them in the evening. Patients will understand such a telephone call as a thoughtful gesture. This is an especially important procedure when husband and wife are both employed. If you are trying to confirm an appointment with a teenager, enlist the assistance of a parent.
2. Many of your patients have dental insurance that provides benefits for dependents. If all benefits are not used within the calendar year, they are lost forever. Write to your insurance patients; encourage them to use all of the benefits to which they are entitled.
3. Most patients, young or old, are interested in cosmetic dentistry. Have you informed all your patients that this is a service available from your practice? Send the fine support material available from the ADA.
4. If a patient, because of chronic illness or age, is unable to visit the office, arrange for a house call. This is a courtesy appreciated by the entire family.
5. Don't forget patients who fail to keep their recare appointments. To do so is an indication on your part that their dental welfare is of no more concern to you than apparently it is to them. If the patient fails to respond to regular recare, let a month or two lapse before

contacting him/her again. Patients are always looking for other ways to spend their money than dentistry. It is important that you prove that dental care is a worthwhile purchase and a wise investment.

6. Remember the 80-20 rule of sales and marketing and apply it to your hygiene department protocol. Only 20% of your patient base will accept your recommendations the first time that you make them. However, a large portion of the remaining 80% *will* begin to comply with your advice on the fourth or fifth encounter.

7. Check the list of patients for whom you provided full and partial dentures more than a year ago. Ask them to return for examination because of the potential of non-discovered cancer.

8. Review the list of inactive patients, those who have not visited you in more than a year, those who have failed to complete planned treatment, and those who have called to postpone an appointment and never rescheduled. Give this list to your most enthusiastic staff member, the one with the most pleasing phone personality. With a record of each patient to guide her conversation, let her emphasize your concern for the patient's dental condition.

9. Reactivate. Reactivate. Reactivate. (Fig. 9-1)

Dear _____,

When you were in our office for your last dental cleaning, we diagnosed early periodontal (gum) disease in your mouth. Our recommendation therapy includes a series of meticulous, thorough "cleanings", specifically designed to remove disease-causing tartar and plaque below the gum line. This procedure leaves a healthy environment around the gums, which can be maintained through good oral hygiene habits.

We are concerned that you have not scheduled your periodontal therapy at this time, and wish to remind you that much of the success of this therapy is based upon treating the condition in its earliest stages.

Unfortunately, gum disease has very few signs or symptoms until it is in the advanced stages. Please call our office to schedule an appointment as soon as possible. _____ will be happy to make your appointment. I will look forward to seeing you soon. Please call me if you have any questions.

Sincerely,

_____

Dear _____,

We've missed you and your bright smile at Dr. _____'s dental practice.

Our records show that it has been _____ months since you've been in. Your continued optimum oral health is of primary concern to us.

We're a prevention-oriented practice and find that routine checkups greatly reduce preventable treatment. Even if you aren't experiencing any discomfort at this time, wouldn't it ease your mind to have a dental professional safely and expertly evaluate your dental needs?

Please contact us for an appointment today. Your dental health is very important.

Sincerely,

_____

Dear _____,

In checking our records recently, we found it has been _____ months since your mouth has been examined. During our recent examination, we found some areas that need treatment. To this date, we have not completed this treatment.

We never want to give dental problems a chance to get ahead of us. At this point, the odds are in your favor that you will not have trouble, provided treatment is completed in a timely manner. Of course, correction of a problem at a later date may be very difficult, more painful, and usually more expensive.

Please call our office today to schedule a 10-minute, no-charge appointment with me to discuss our concerns for your oral care.

Sincerely,

_____

Figure 9–1 Sample Reactivation Letters

Dear _____,

In a recent review of our records, we have found that your last dental visit with us was quite some time ago. In our effort to provide the most comprehensive care for our patients, we feel it is necessary to contact you with this letter. We are concerned that you have not been receiving necessary dental care, such as regular periodontal evaluations for the prevention of gum disease. Six-month dental check-ups are also important for the detection of dental decay, broken fillings, and any additional problems you might be having. We automatically provide complete preventive exams for the detection of oral cancer. We hope to hear from you soon, so that we may keep your records active in our preventive care program.

Yours for better health,

_____

Dear _____,

In a recent review of our records, we have found that your last dental visit with us was _____ months ago. In our effort to provide the most comprehensive care for our patients, we feel it necessary to contact you with this letter. We miss you _____ and are concerned that you are receiving necessary dental care, such as regular periodontal evaluations for the prevention of gum disease. Six-month dental check-ups are also important for the detection dental decay, broken fillings, and any additional problems you might be having. We automatically provide complete preventive exams for the detection of oral cancer.

We hope to hear from you soon so that we may keep your records active in our preventive care program. Should you have an emergency, we can be reached by our 24-hour answering service to provide you with prompt dental care.

Yours for better health,

_____

Figure 9–1 continued

CURING THE BLACK HOLE SYNDROME
THROUGH CHART AUDITING

*Great works are performed not by
strength, but by perseverance.*
— SAMUEL JOHNSON

All dental professionals should keep two goals in mind: clinical excellence and management excellence. While most dentists are diligent about the first, too few pay adequate attention to the second. Many dentists, for example, mistakenly feel that the only way to increase practice profitability is to get more and more new patients. Some spend thousands of dollars implementing expensive external marketing plans to achieve this goal, never noticing that as new patients arrive at the front door, an equal or greater flow of patients is walking out the back door. These patients' records fall into a seemingly bottomless black hole.

This black hole syndrome can be more costly than most dental professionals realize. Every patient who disappears from a dental practice represents an unrealized treatment program, an untapped cosmetic or restorative procedure, or a lost potential source for new patient referrals.

Fortunately, an antidote exists. It can be found on the shelves of an out-of-the-way closet or in the dusty filing cabinets sitting somewhere behind last year's Christmas decorations. It is in these forgotten corners that every dental practice keeps its dead practice files, the secret and untapped acres of diamonds that have lain dormant for a year or more. Mining these acres of diamonds, like real diamond mining, is admittedly a tedious procedure. The rewards, as in real diamond mining, can be enormous and are well worth the effort.

Thousands of dollars of recommended preventive and restorative treatment can come from reactivating practice files, and the process begins with an aggressive chart audit. The technique is simple. The first thing to do is to pull the files A to Z and see why the people attached to those files got lost. Perhaps they missed a scheduled appointment; perhaps no follow up appointment was ever scheduled. Audit out at two years (24 months). These files are removed from the main file storage area and placed somewhere else. We can come back to them. Then begin to check from 23 months to the present time. Patients absent for 11 months or less can be called. Patients absent longer than 11 months can be sent a reactivation letter.

The premise behind the reactivation program is to identify and recapture three types of patients:

- those who have not returned for their preventive, continuing care appointments
- those who were presented with diagnosis and a treatment plan but have not completed treatment
- those who were diagnosed but not presented with a treatment plan

It is important to assess what went on during that last office visit and determine what a logical follow-up visit should have been about. What happened, for example, to Mrs. Smith, who seemed so excited about having some empress inlays placed? What about little Suzy, whose mother promised to schedule for sealants once the school year ended? What about Mr. Jones, who seemed so interested in the periodontal program we discussed with him when he called to complain about his bleeding gums?

When orchestrating the auditing campaign, it is imperative to make sure that the process be consistent, organized, and very polished. Deciding before-hand who will do what can defuse potential disagreements before they occur. Deciding how many files to audit a day, a week, and a month establishes specific goals that are easier to achieve than ambiguous goals. Successful chart auditing may require scheduling adjustments, and this should be part of the master plan. It may also require making judgment calls on certain issues. How many times, for example, should a patient be contacted for reactivation purposes? Will offering a free consultation make reactivation more likely? Is this cost effective? Thus, before jumping into the campaign you must answer the following questions:

1. Who will do the audit?
2. What diagnostic information will we look for?
3. Who will make the calls?
4. Who will mail the letters?
5. How many files do we want to audit a day, a week, and a month?

6. Will we monitor the patients leaving and why?
7. Will we do an exit interview when necessary?
8. What time of the day will be for auditing?
9. Will we do free consultations with reactivated patients?
10. How many times should we contact the patient to obtain an appointment?

You will also need to train your chart auditing team to look for certain key information:

1. When was the last recare visit?
2. What was the last treatment completed?
3. Are any insurance claims unattended?
4. Is medical history complete?
5. Are medical alerts designated?
6. Is all necessary information on registration form completed satisfactorily?
7. Have you charted existing restorations?
8. What type and size are existing restorations?
9. Was full probing done?
10. Were recession, bleeding points, furcation involvement, mobility, occlusal discrepancies, and fremitus properly charted?
11. Was any periodontal treatment recommended? If so, what type and why?
12. What was case presented?
13. What did the patient accept?
14. Were finances discussed?
15. Are there additional notes or comments in the file that will assist you in reactivating the patient?

Keeping accurate records of chart auditing activities is a must, especially if several staff members are involved in the process.

Making the follow up visit happen is the next logical step. There should be a meaningful phone call from the practice, with the caller expressing concern for the person, not just the person's dental work. It is always best to contact patients by phone and follow up with a letter. Since it can cost approximately $7 to mail a letter, each letter should be proactive, convincing, and inviting.

What really affects whether or not the audit is successful is the team's ability to communicate with the patients effectively and win them over so they reactivate themselves back into the practice. The old saying "It's not what you say, but how you say it, that is so important" is the basis of completing a successful chart audit. You must script excellently and then continue to practice with your staff until the message you want to deliver is perfectly orchestrated every time. There are several useful scripts you can incorporate into your practice protocol:

Reactivation call

Mrs. Smith, This is Cindy from Dr. Jones' office. Dr. Jones has reviewed your file and expressed concern to me that we have not seen you in our office for your preventive maintenance appointment in almost two years. We know that you want to keep your teeth a lifetime. Preventive dental care will ensure this. I would like to schedule an appointment for you with our hygienist, Sue. Which day would be best for you and do you prefer a.m. or p.m.?

Patient responds, "I can't make an appointment now, I'm too busy."

"I understand Mrs. Smith, I'll just jot a note to Dr. Jones stating that it is just not a good time for you. I would like to contact you again within the next few months. Would October or November work for you?"

Patient responds, "I'm not coming back to the practice."

"Mrs. Smith, I am so sorry to hear that you will not be returning to our practice. We have really enjoyed having you as part of our family of patients. Please keep in mind that our office is only a telephone call away. Our team continues to work on improving ourselves. If you wouldn't mind sharing, what can we do to improve our service to our patients?"

Exit interview - formal

"Dr. Jones and his team are very committed to providing our patients with excellence in quality dentistry and care. We welcome feedback, be it positive or negative. Would you share with me what our practice could do to improve our delivery of care to our patients? Could I ask you why you are seeking care somewhere else? Mrs. Smith, if the next practice you go to does not provide the

quality of care you've been receiving here, we want you to know our door is always open to you."

Patient unhappy with the dentistry we've done

Mrs. Smith, I am so happy I've contacted you. I hope you will let us have an opportunity to remedy this situation. Dr. Jones would want me to schedule an appointment with him for a consultation. What day and time a.m. or p.m. works for you?"

Keep the patient files available for a future team meeting for review of inactive patients. Keep a monthly log and then an annual log of patients leaving the practice and why they are leaving. The documentation will provide extremely useful information showing the trends and possible patterns that are developing in your practice's acres of diamonds. You then can develop an appropriate action plan that is used by the team to turn weaknesses into opportunities.

Of course, there are going to be patients we choose not to approach during a reactivation audit. Among these are patients who have been designated not to contact, those who are collection problems, those who have left the practice because they have switched to a capitation plan, or those who are generally not solicited for other reasons.

BROKEN APPOINTMENTS AND HOW TO FIX THEM

National statistics show that dental practices lose approximately 15% of their patients somewhere between scheduling and production. The entire 15% comes from broken appointments, cancellations, and no shows. Broken appointments can cost the average practice up to $40,000 a year. In most instances, the broken appointment represents not only a lost fee, but loss of productivity. The hour or so scheduled with the patient who did not come can never truly be recovered.

Some practices attempt to resolve the problem by taking punitive measures. Dentists charge a total or partial fee for missed appointments and feel they have not really lost out. Unfortunately, studies confirm that this approach is not only ineffective, but can be quite counter-productive. Almost invariably, patients view it as an unfair over-reaction. For some, being charged for time they were not in the office is more than sufficient grounds for leaving a practice altogether.

A far better way to deal with the problem of broken appointments is to establish a proactive office policy that is designed to minimize their number. This means letting all patients know that your time is too valuable to waste. Patients who break appointments by simply not showing up do not understand this at all. Every one of these patients needs to be told, or reminded, that you expect a phone call if an appointment cannot be kept. Put this message in your brochures and on all correspondence, bills, or reminder postcards sent to patients. Train your appointment coordinator and your hygienist and your billing clerk to deliver this message clearly and frequently, especially to those patients who have a record of blowing off appointments without notice.

You are slightly ahead of the game if patients who break appointments call before doing so, but not by much. Consider the following. When patients call to cancel or reschedule an appointment, they obviously disrupt the schedule for the day of the appointment. What is less obvious is the disruption they cause the day they call. The receptionist or front desk staff member is taken away from other duties and must spend valuable (and unbillable) time discussing the situation with the patient and finding a suitable date and time to schedule a new visit. This conversation may take up to 10 minutes. More time must be spent calling other patients in hopes that one of them may opt to come in and fill in that "unexpected opening."

There are many reason patients give for breaking appointments, but most fall into three categories: legitimate, creative but suspect, or bogus and chronic.

The legitimate reason is usually straightforward and easy to spot. It comes from the patient who is generally conscientious, keeps appointments diligently, comes on time, and has a healthy financial relationship with the practice. When this patient calls to cancel, you can assume the problem is real. The patient is usually sincerely apologetic and quick to suggest that the appointment be rescheduled as soon as possible. This patient may even be open to suggestions that might make keeping the appointment possible – alternative transportation or baby-sitting arrangements.

"Creative but suspect" excuses are another matter altogether. These come from patients who *can* come but are calling because they *do not want* to come. Invariably, these patients believe in visiting a dental practice, but not too much. They want to come when something is a problem and usually show up for that annual cleaning, but they are not especially interested in anything else. They may agree to treatment programs or to routine periodontal examinations, but sooner or later the regular visits become tedious and disagreeable, and the calls to cancel or reschedule come more frequently. Their philosophy boils down to "if it ain't broke, don't fix it, and if it doesn't hurt, it ain't broke."

These patients do not fully understand the value of excellent dentistry. Simply put, they have not been properly educated, and the first task at hand is to make sure that this situation is rectified. A dentist or hygienist needs to explain clearly and precisely any existing problems, any potential problems, and any and all consequences of leaving problems untreated. Preventive dentistry should be clearly explained; compliance should be reinforced.

With these patients, a call breaking an appointment should never be encouraged. The receptionist should sound friendly, but disappointed. A happy-sounding or even neutral response suggests that breaking appointments is acceptable. Front desk staff must never make it easy for these patients to cancel. Any excuse should be countered with a potential solution:

"I'm sorry to hear about your car, Mr. Jones. What time would you like us to send a cab for you?"

"I'll be happy to watch the baby for you during your appointment. Babies sleep 18 hours a day and she'll probably sleep the whole time. It's no bother at all."

Few of us can claim that we have never used "illness" as an excuse to skip a test in school, to extend a weekend away from work, or to get out of an unappealing social engagement. Dentists might hear this "creative but suspect" excuse less frequently by trying the following script. "I'm sorry you have a cold, but if you feel well enough to come in, please do. Dr. Smith can use a mask and gloves and we've all had our flu shots this year." If the patient insists she is too sick to make it to the office, a get well card, signed by the entire staff, should be sent.

Make it clear to the members of the "creative but suspect" crew that rescheduling an appointment is a complicated and time-consuming imposition. You should never be rude, but playing "if you can't beat 'em join 'em" is quite acceptable—a little well-placed whining can be very effective. Above all, never make it easy and never have exactly the time they want available. The message will come across loud and clear.

The bogus and chronic appointment-breaker seldom has a good excuse and frequently has no excuse at all. It is perfectly acceptable to confront such a patient and call a spade a spade. Say politely but firmly, "We seem to be having a problem coordinating your busy schedule with ours. We're making a note in your chart that you will call us with a date you can definitely be here and that we will then coordinate your appointment time with ours." The patient has made irresponsible decisions that have upset your schedule and your productivity. Now you have made the entire appointment scheduling process the patient's responsibility. The patient may surprise you and rise to the challenge; he or she is most likely to live up to your expectations and completely disappear from the practice. With the chronic excuse patient, either scenario is preferable to having you schedule appointments that are sure to be broken.

Some general recommendations for reducing the number of broken appointments can be applied to all patients. Showing patients that you value their time makes it more likely that they will value yours. Calling to tell a patient "We're looking forward to seeing you tomorrow" is much better than "calling to remind." Sending appointment confirmation cards for appointments made months in advance is a good idea. The cards should say "we will see you on the 20th", not "call us if this time is not convenient." Making the entire practice staff aware of the havoc broken appointments wreak on productivity and profitability makes the entire staff more likely to treat the problem seriously and proactively.

Pearls to Reduce Cancellations and Broken Appointments

- The doctor and the entire staff should discuss the perils of lost time. Schedule a team meeting to review your monitors of the unscheduled hours. The hours turned into dollars per hour lost can be quite extensive. Becoming aware of the issues makes them much easier to alleviate. Review these issues at least quarterly with the entire team.
- Value patients' time so that they will learn to value yours. Being prompt to see patients conveys that "I am valued here!" Patients will respect your time to the same degree that their time is respected.
- Write office protocol for patients who habitually break appointments. (Fig. 9-2) After several broken appointments without a good excuse, say, "We seem to be having a problem coordinating your busy schedule with ours. Is there a concern about the treatment plan we have designed for you, Mrs. Smith? We're making a note in your clinical record that you will call us with a date you can definitely be here so that we can coordinate your appointment time with ours."
- Role-play the verbiage and remember that practice makes perfect. Role-playing once a month can give the entire dental team an added edge with their verbal skills. In addition, makes sure everyone is talking the same talk.
- Educate patients about the value of their "reserved" time when the appointment is made. Using the word "reserved" makes an appointment sound more important and a patient will be more apt to keep it.
- Sound disappointed, yet friendly when patients try to change or break appointments. A happy-sounding or neutral response indicates it is not only alright to fail to keep the appointment, but also totally acceptable. Without sounding rude or abrupt, a good appointment secretary displays friendly concern and disappointment at the same time.
- Offer workable solutions to the problems patients have in not keeping scheduled appointments. When the appointment becomes important to you, it will become important to your patients.

- Confirm by mail all appointments that are scheduled months in advance. Make sure the message is positive instead of, "if this time is not convenient, please call for another appointment."
- Do not call to "remind" patients. Say, "We're looking forward to seeing you tomorrow."
- Send get well cards (signed by the entire team) to patients who use the excuse that they are ill.
- Make the rescheduling opportunity very difficult. If the patient finds out that there is not another appointment for "at least three weeks," and "I know that the hygienist or dentist does not want you to wait that long," patients may be more apt to keep the scheduled appointment.
- Finally, have a quick call list (consisting of patients who do not appoint each time) to fill holes in the schedule the moment they happen.

Mr. John Forgetter
1818 Main Street
Any town, USA 10050

Dear Mr. Forgetter:

On January 30, February 12, and March 10, you failed to keep your appointments at my office. In my opinion, your condition requires continued dental treatment. If you so desire, you may telephone our office for another appointment, but if you prefer to have another dentist attend you, I suggest that you arrange to do so without delay. You may be assured that, at your request, I am entirely willing to make available my knowledge of your case to the dentist of your choice.

I trust that you will understand that my purpose in writing this letter is out of concern for your health and well being.

Sincerely,

I. M. Caring, DDS

Figure 9–2 Letter to Patient Who Fails to Keep Multiple Appointments

WATCHING THE BACK DOOR

Much effort, much prosperity.
— EURIPIDES

Long-term success for a dental practice is dependent on the commitment of repeat, loyal patients. Unfortunately, statistical evidence on patient commitment and loyalty to a dental practice is quite disconcerting. Nationwide, the life span of a dental patient's visit to the same practice is only three years. The average practice will lose approximately 10% of its patients through attrition each year. Every month, 20% of the patients scheduled for appointments change or cancel their appointments or simply fail to show up. The average dental practice in the United States maintains less than a 50% recare effectiveness percentage monthly and annually. An extrapolation of these numbers indicates that the average dental practice experiences a 50% patient turnover every five years.

These startling statistics can bring any dental business to its knees. Trying to find the magic curative formula, dental practitioners invest thousands of dollars on elaborate marketing campaigns and new technology in the belief that these will increase their productivity and profitability. Team members feel that if they look better or show off a beautiful computer or fancy optical loupes, patients will be so impressed with them, they will never leave the office to go elsewhere. New patient lists are closely monitored each month for numbers and for referral sources. A strategy to increase efforts to market to these sources with more repetition and vigor is rigorously implemented. With so much attention focused on the front door, too few offices pay enough attention to the back door. Too little time is spent monitoring patients who don't come back, and even less time is spent on discovering why they don't come back and formulating a policy to prevent this from happening.

There are many reasons patients leave dental practices. Some are beyond our control; others are very much within the range of our control, and concerted efforts can and should be made to ensure retention. A recent statistical analysis compiled by the American Dental Association cites the following information on why patients leave dental practices:

- 1% die
- 2% move away
- 4% are chronic complainers who find fault with all service-oriented professions and therefore maintain ties with all service-oriented professionals only before moving on to others
- 5% change to dental practices recommended by friends
- 7% change because they have found a practice that charges lower fees
- 17% change because of insurance company constraints that limit coverage for certain services or limit coverage to a restricted list of practices
- 64% go elsewhere because they are dissatisfied

We have absolutely no control over patients who die or move away. This group, however, represents only 3% of the patients our practices lose each year. The 4% group of chronic complainers who don't like anybody very much is, to a certain extent, also beyond anyone's control, and investing time and energy in retaining patients of this ilk may be more trouble than it is worth. Patients in this group are generally difficult to deal with, potentially disruptive to the practice schedule, and can do the practice more harm than good in terms of marketing and public relations aimed at attracting new patients.

This leaves a rather hefty group of patients (93%) that leave practices for reasons ranging from financial issues to customer dissatisfaction. Almost invariably, these reasons can be challenged—they represent circumstances that truly are within our control.

Those patients who leave for purportedly financial reasons represent 24% of the total number of patients changing dental practices. The 7% who leave because they have found practices that deliver dental care that is cheaper have not been properly educated about value. What we have in this instance is dental fees that are being challenged as too high or even exorbitant. Patients who choose practices charging lower fees many not realize that they may be short-changing themselves. While we do not mean to imply that lower fees mean lower standards of quality, fees do sometimes reflect the difference between the number and type of services offered. They can also reflect a difference in the level of technology to which an office has access, technology that frequently makes a significant difference to patients in clinical evaluations and in treatment procedures. Lower or higher fees can also be attributed to anesthetics—painless, comfortable dentistry has its price. In many cases, patients are aware only of the bottom line. They do not realize, unless we tell them, what they many be losing in the transition.

Patients who leave a practice because of restrictive insurance company regulations (17%) are also salvageable. While managed health care represents a challenge to all medical and dental practitioners, it is a challenge that can be confronted from several directions. If your practice is not on the "approved" list of a patient's insurance carrier, steps can be taken to have your practice added to this list. If procedures you recommend as necessary and important to a patient's oral health are questioned, and payment for these procedures does not qualify for coverage, steps can also be taken to counter the carriers' arguments for non-payment or low partial payment. In both cases, it may be necessary to enlist the assistance of patients, who should be encouraged to question and even protest insurance company policies. It is also essential to let patients know that the insurance companies' decisions on treatment procedures are not always in patients' best interests, whereas your ethical commitment to their well being is. Here again, education on the value of preventive dentistry and routine visits for oral health maintenance can make a tremendous difference.

A full 69% of patients leaving dental practices leave because they are dissatisfied customers. Five percent of these go to practices recommended by friends or acquaintances. It is more than likely that these recommendations are not the underlying reason patients leave—they are merely the end result. Happy, satisfied patients do not leave a practice just because someone else suggests it is a good idea. If, however, a patient complains about a dental practice, a dentist, or a hygienist, someone satisfied with his own or her own dental practice will invariably present a good case for that patient to come aboard. It is at this juncture that all of us should ask ourselves why those patients didn't like our practice enough to encourage other patients dissatisfied with other practices to join ours.

At any rate, we need to examine the reasons 69% of our patients are unhappy enough to leave our practices. Nine out of ten patients will tell you that they judge quality not by how well you prep a crown or scale a tooth. The average patient judges quality on a less concrete and less tangible scale of measurement. What matters most is the "whole experience" they have in your practice. Technical excellence or quality, from the patient's point of view, accounts for 20% of that. The other 80% is based on the intangible and sometimes indefinable "feel good" factor.

All of this boils down to customer service. In many parts of the world, people settle for a service or product that may not be excellent or even adequate. They take what they can get because there are no alternatives. In America, quality customer service is an essential component to business success. This is a two-edged sword. As consumers, we all benefit from living in a country where our choices are virtually limitless. As professionals, we must understand that our businesses survive, succeed, and thrive only when we understand and live by this economic principle.

Almost half of U.S. businesses are service related. Customers patronize certain services and avoid others. Quality products are a must, but customers judge a business on other criteria as well. Customers want to be treated well, and businesses that emphasize good personal service bring customers back and keep them.

In dentistry, as in other service-related fields, business survival depends on maintaining a competitive edge. For this reason, more and more dental practices are working on improving their customer service skills. Expanding the patient base is important, but it should never be limited to attracting new patients. The lifeblood of a practice is repeat, loyal patients who can be our best allies in getting those new patients to come through the front door. Quality service makes this happen. It is the most important ingredient in the mix of things that can keep a patient from saying, "A dentist is a dentist is a dentist"!

No one in a master dental practice ever forgets that dentistry is a business. Every employee in such a practice recognizes that the customer truly is the boss. Everyone in the practice knows that a satisfied customer comes back and a dissatisfied customer doesn't. Everyone in the practice strives to make every patient comfortable, both physically and emotionally. To do this effectively, every member of the dental team must become a student of human behavior. Each must learn to read accurately:

- What the customer wants
- What the customer needs
- What the customer thinks
- What the customer feels
- Whether the customer is satisfied
- Whether the customer is planning to return

Once we realize that there is really a body with feelings attached to that mouth, we begin to empathize. Empathy means putting ourselves in patients' shoes and viewing a situation through their eyes. It means realizing that these multiple appointments in the operatory chair are not only time consuming but stressful, scary, and costly. We must ask ourselves, "If I were this person, what would I want?"

All patients have four basic desires and our successes are dependent on our ability to satisfy these:

- Need to be understood
- Need to feel welcome
- Need to feel important
- Need to be comfortable

Keeping the customer's needs and wants satisfied requires a commitment and discipline. It means we must resolutely and consistently practice the following:

- Always being pleasant to patients even if they are not pleasant to us
- Welcoming patients' suggestions on how the practice can improve its services
- Graciously listening to and handling any complaints or problems
- Smiling even when we don't feel like smiling
- Rolling with the punches and turning on a dime
- Providing service that is above and beyond the call of duty (and above and beyond what the competitor has to offer)
- Thoroughly and enthusiastically explaining the features and benefits of all of the dental services provided by the practice
- Projecting sincerity and compassion to every patient.
- Calling patients after major therapy
- Responding quickly to patients' concerns
- Making patient comfort a priority
- Working quickly and efficiently
- Greeting patients by name
- Escorting patient to the door after a visit
- Providing a mirror so a patient can "freshen up" before leaving the operatory
- Ensuring that the only background noise is soothing music
- Seeing patients punctually

- Sending new patients welcome packets before their appointment with a handwritten note from the dentist
- Providing a variety of payment options
- Offering senior citizens courtesy discounts

A management strategy beyond improving relationships with patients and incorporating customer service techniques is the use of a patient satisfaction survey. Consider the following survey, pre-folded, and stuffed in self-addressed, stamped envelopes randomly presented to selected patients every month. (Fig. 9-3) One person in the office should be given the responsibility of compiling the responses. A portion of the monthly staff meeting should be devoted to a review of new patients and their referral source, a review of the survey information, and a review of patients' suggestions on how the practice can improve its service.

We hope that you have had a comfortable and pleasant experience in our office. We would greatly appreciate it if you would take a moment to share your impressions of our practice. We are always striving to be the best that we can.

A = Excellent   B = Average   C = Could be improved

1. Friendliness of staff	A	B	C
2. Scheduling of appointments worked for you	A	B	C
3. The front team members were courteous and helpful	A	B	C
4. Treatment consultations were comprehensive	A	B	C
5. We were on time for you	A	B	C
6. Front desk personnel were professional and courteous	A	B	C
7. Courteousness and concern of chair-side assistants	A	B	C
8. Doctor was helpful and knowledgeable	A	B	C
9. Dental hygienists were knowledgeable and courteous	A	B	C
10. Chair-side assistants were gentle	A	B	C
11. Hygienists were gentle	A	B	C
12. Doctor was gentle	A	B	C
13. Reception room was comfortable	A	B	C
14. Treatment area was clean and attractive	A	B	C
15. All your questions were answered to your satisfaction	A	B	C
16. The quality of our service	A	B	C
17. The value of the services we provide	A	B	C
18. Would you recommend our office to your friends?	Yes	No	

19. Do you have any comments that would help us to improve our service to you?

_____

_____

_____

Figure 9–3 Commitment to Excellence

Even with all of these components in place, there is no guarantee that something wasn't missed somewhere and some patients will still choose to leave your practice. Minimizing the number of patients who take this road means learning why some have chosen to do so. It is important, therefore, to monitor the patients leaving the practice and the reasons why they are leaving. Keep an updated log and report the number during team meetings. Make sure to relate the number to the new patient final numbers each month so you can determine whether or not the practice is in a positive, flat, or negative growth mode. List the reasons patients are leaving and list them in order of priority. When more than one response continues to appear, it becomes increasing more apparent that the practice has a problem that must be adjusted. Do not ignore even the most inane reasons given. Old magazines in the waiting area may not seem very important to you, but it may truly be one patient's reason for leaving.

Our patients are the only reason we report to our practices on a daily, monthly and annual basis. They are the only commodity we have. By taking responsibility for watching the back door, we take active steps toward improving our practice immeasurably. When this occurs, our patients will stop walking out the back door. Indeed, they will become the single best form of advertisement for bringing new patients in the front door.

10 Scheduling for the Practice and the Pulse of the Practice

OBJECTIVES OF SCHEDULING

There never was yet philosopher that
could endure the toothache patiently.
— WILLIAM SHAKESPEARE

Even under the best circumstances, no patient truly wants to be in a dental office. Some deal with it better than others, but if we are to be honest with ourselves, we know this is an absolute given. We all know that patients prefer to visit a dental office as few times as possible. They want to come in at 8 a.m. and be out at 9 a.m. or come in at 4 p.m. and be out at 5 p.m. with all of their work completed during one office visit. They want to be seen promptly and have all work done quickly and painlessly and without delay or interruption. Unfortunately, this ideal scenario is very difficult to find in most dental practices. What really happens is quite different.

To begin with, there is no consistency. Some days, everyone's needs are met and everything goes as planned. Goals are reached and there are no surprises. On other days, everything goes wrong. Patients are seen late, treatment is not completed, and every delay seems to breed new delays. By the end of the day, little has been accomplished and the whole team feels exhausted. Patients see a dental team that seems disorganized and uncoordinated. This is bad for everyone and is the main reason a master dental practice needs to have an effective scheduling policy.

No patient wants to sit around in the reception area waiting to be seen. No patient likes sitting in an operatory chair while the dentist or hygienist is off in another room washing up, changing gloves, looking for files or x-rays or instruments, or doing something else while the anesthetic is taking effect. Patients left waiting around are patients who feel that their time is being wasted. This perception of wasted time is one of the chief complaints patients have about their dental practices. An effective scheduling policy can eliminate a great deal of the waiting time that makes patients feel this way. It also provides a stress-free environment for the dental team. It gives a structure to each day that ensures stability rather than chaos. Establishing a good scheduling policy also helps improve production efficiency.

Thus, the objectives of scheduling must include the following components:

- Taking care of patient needs
- Providing a stress-free environment for everyone
- Making certain production goals are met

None of this can happen without a plan. These three objectives can be met by incorporating block scheduling into your daily routine. In this program, the staff decides what works well on successful days and duplicates it every day. Once established, the blocks do not change from day to day. This will take a great deal of discipline and skill on the part of the entire dental team.

PRODUCTION EFFICIENCY AND SCHEDULING: DETERMINING WHERE YOU ARE AND WHERE YOU NEED TO BE

Production efficiency is one of those areas most often dominated by and defined by tradition and inertia. Things are kept where they have always been kept; things are done the way they have always been done. In a master practice, this is unacceptable. Careful attention to time and design is a must.

- Is the office designed for effective movement of patients?
- Is anything causing a delay?
- Is treatment provided on schedule?
- Do we do unscheduled procedures that can cause unacceptable delays in the day's schedule?
- Do we regularly run on time?
- Does everyone arrive on time?
- Do we have a morning huddle to discuss potential delays and solutions?

Time is important to everyone. In a master practice, time means paying attention to *scheduling*. An efficient system will take into account all contingencies and all potential problems. There should also be a standard protocol for dealing with these. To determine whether scheduling should be an area of concern in your practice, review the following:

- Are recare (recall) appointments pre-appointed?
- Is there an effective filing system that minimizes filing and retrieval time?
- Do scheduling techniques track the doctor *and* the hygienist?
- Do we block too much time for certain procedures?
- Do we block insufficient time for certain procedures?
- Do we monitor failed or late appointments?
- Do we schedule time for emergencies?
- Do we run on time?
- Do we schedule certain procedures at specific times? Is this office policy?
- Are separate appointment books used for the dentist *and* the hygienist?
- Is the team consulted about scheduling concerns, issues, problems, and solutions?

SCHEDULING WITHOUT CHAOS

*I must govern the clock, not be
governed by it.* – GOLDA MEIR

Many dental practices seem to schedule their appointment books by filling in the lines. Teams panic when there is white space in the appointment book or when they see a computerized scheduler without a name. Quickly they put anything into the schedule. This ends up producing a day with emergencies, no lunch, running behind, low production, no-shows, and a lot of stress. It goes without saying that the practice probably did not reach the goal for the day. Everyone on the team is tired, worn out, and probably looking for a new job.

Dental practices can reach their daily, monthly, and annual scheduling and production goals two ways: qualitatively and quantitatively. The master dental practice always commits itself to reaching scheduling and production goals qualitatively, by looking at the types of procedures being scheduled in the dental chair and not the number of patients in the dental chair.

Currently available to dental professionals are hundreds of manuals that purport to teach us hundreds of ways to schedule a profitable day. Some have good ideas; others do not. Careful research of over 500 dental practices nationwide provides evidence that implementing certain "golden guidelines" will consistently bring the dental practice and team stress-free, productive, ideal days. The first of these guidelines is choosing a designated driver.

Many dental practices have a front desk patient care coordinator. This is a person who must be skilled in time management. It is her function to make each day run smoothly. Her job description includes updating patient forms, confirming appointments, welcoming new patients, distributing brochures and business cards, filling in the holes in the schedule by placing well-timed calls to patients who may be interested in time-slots unexpectedly left open, sending recare promotion letters, sending personal notes, and making reactivation calls.

It takes extensive training to help someone with dental knowledge to learn to schedule productively. The person handling the schedule must be able to think in terms of scheduling toward the daily goal. By listening to other team members, learning from experience, and by studying the numbers, she should be able to schedule ideal days—income per hour between $300 and $400 for the doctor and between $100 and $150 per hour for the hygienist. She should help monitor hygiene statistics to determine whether the office is achieving 85% or better recare effectiveness. When time permits, this person should be actively involved in chart auditing and re-activation activities. To accomplish all of these functions, she needs to communicate regularly and productively with the doctor and the hygienist, and this means that she must actively participate in team meetings and the morning huddle during which crucial scheduling issues are discussed.

In practices grossing under $30,000 per month, there is usually only one person at the front desk. We have seen practices without a front desk person; in these practices, the assistants or hygienists maintain the front desk activity as they can. Usually, these practices are in total chaos, are very low-procedure, and are poorly structured. Without a "quarterback," it is difficult to run the team. In a practice grossing in excess of $40,000 per month, there should be a special person to see that each professional is booked productively. That person's primary responsibility is to construct as perfect a day as possible within the guidelines set forth by the team.

The patient care coordinator's work is simplified if specific guidelines are in place for scheduling activities if the appointment book is used, and the same would impact computer scheduling:

1. Use a pencil or computer.
2. Use full name of patient. Designate age of child.
3. Write in home as well as work phone numbers.
4. Designate medical alerts.
5. Use abbreviations for welfare patients, reduced fee patients, new patients, or emergency patients.
6. Designate the tooth number, procedure, and material to be used. (i.e., #14 MOD, composite).
7. Designate the dollar amount of the procedure.
8. Track the chair time with a straight line.
9. Track the total doctor time to the right or left of the schedule.

10. *Hygiene appointments are scheduled in a separate appointment book.* (Very important!)
11. Fill hard-to-schedule times first.
12. If appointment schedules are computerized, maintain the computer and practice computer safety rules. Back up diligently.

Another useful tool for the patient care coordinator is a patient call list, which can be used to confirm appointments, to fill spaces left by cancellations, and for re-activation projects. An example follows (Fig. 10-1).

Date	Name	Adress or Telephone	Service Requested	Time Preferred	Notified

Figure 10—1 Patient Call List

Scheduling and the Hygienist: an Alternative

In most dental practices, scheduling patient appointments is purely a front-desk function. In the case of new patients or old patients who call for an appointment because there is a problem, this is fine. In the case of recare appointments, however, it is far more efficient to make scheduling the responsibility of the dental hygienist. This has manifold benefits. Scheduling an appointment at the front desk is scheduling an appointment with someone who is not directly involved with a patient's care. If the dental hygienist and the patient have achieved a good relationship, the patient is likely to be comfortable knowing that the hygienist is scheduling a "personal" appointment for follow up care.

The hygienist can more accurately gauge than can the front desk team member the amount of time a recare visit with a particular patient will take. In scheduling an appointment, she can set up a realistic block of time and thus avoid the problem of having a patient sitting around in the waiting room while she finishes with another patient. It also gives the hygienist more control over flextime. Down time created by holes in front desk scheduling is not always efficient; down time or flex time deliberately built into a weekly or daily schedule so that dental hygienist can attend to tasks not directly related to seeing patients is purposeful and meaningful.

Scheduling for Productivity: Setting and Achieving Goals

Most busy offices see far too many people per day. This causes an excessive amount of work by auxiliaries both in the front office and the operatory area. In the treatment area, large numbers of patients create extensive set up and aseptic procedures. The common characteristics of "ideal" days are as follows:

- Fewer patients are treated.
- A large amount of treatment is accomplished for each patient.
- Appointments are on time.
- Time is allotted to handle emergencies.
- A quiet, relaxed atmosphere prevails.
- Goals are reached.

What does a good day in dentistry look like from a scheduling standpoint?

- Quadrant dentistry is scheduled as much as possible.
- The atmosphere of the practice is very relaxed and fun.
- Goals are reached consistently each day.
- Every patient leaves the practice after an appointment the same way: another appointment is scheduled for something, financial arrangements are completed, and two or three business cards are given to each patient to share with friends.

Scheduling the ideal day means determining a daily goal. The dentist and team decide what their ideal day should look like. A daily goal for scheduling is determined. For the dentist, we always want to schedule and produce approximately $300 to $400 per hour. When we speak of engineering an "ideal day," it simply means that we schedule a creative day for the dentist and hygienist that have many different types of procedures, piggybacked off the highest production therapies. In the dentist's chair, the procedures would be crown and bridge and for the hygienist, periodontal root planing. Give priority to productive procedures and don't clutter the appointment book with patch, drill, and fill procedures.

A good day would be if the dentist has scheduled four crown procedures in the morning from 8 to noon. Around lunch, two hours of restorative dentistry should be scheduled, leaving the end of the day from 3 to 5 with the non-productive procedures, such as cement crowns, denture adjustments, and consultations. Booking non-productive procedures should always be accelerated off the primary dentistry or scheduled in the 3 to 5 time blocks, if the practice has enough support staff.

The question of how many operatories a practitioner really needs often arises. We have seen one doctor gross upwards of $1 million with only one operatory for him and one for the hygienist, but this is rare. We believe a doctor can produce on any level he or she chooses with two properly trained assistants and two identical, fully equipped operatories. The doctor then determines how many hygiene operatories are desired—two, perhaps three, operatories, depending on whether the doctor desires the hygienist to do soft tissue management and how far he or she he wishes to carry periodontal patients. All of this must be factored into setting and scheduling for production goals.

All production goals should be practical, reasonable, and attainable. It takes all these attributes for a practice to increase productivity 25 to 30% annually. In fact, a master practice can realistically expect to experience 10 to 30% growth just with proper scheduling and appointment control. The entire group should do this at a team planning session. Review the calendar for the coming year. Once you work with your numbers, see what the practice really produces in a day, and then what is required by the hour, you can begin to set your sight on proper, productive scheduling.

Each day should begin with a 20-minute huddle to review every patient scheduled, troubleshoot for any problems, review how the previous day went, and discuss how tomorrow is shaping up. The morning huddle lets the doctor and hygienist know if they are on target for achieving the practice goals. It also aids in eliminating a great deal of chaos. Everyone should be there.

KNOW HOW MUCH TIME TO ALLOW FOR EACH PROCEDURE

Frequently, a doctor will allow 60 minutes for a restoration and completion, finish in 40 minutes, then waste the remaining 20 minutes. Or the doctor will allow 30 minutes for a procedure and spend 60 minutes doing it. The same time lapses occur in hygiene operatories. The best way to eliminate this problem is to determine the actual amount of time needed for procedures. Use a stopwatch and keep a record for two months on every procedure.

Each time study should cover every detail of a patient's visit. Every procedure, for example, must include doctor time, hygienist time, assistant time, and clean-up time. Break down in exact detail, on the appointment page, the time needed for each procedure performed. Knowing what production time must be per hour helps the doctor establish a proper fee schedule and helps decide what procedures are non-productive and need to be referred. For example, a young doctor establishes that it takes $105 an hour to reach his productivity goal. His fee for a procedure is $250. It takes a total of three hours to complete this procedure. He clearly does not meet his goal. Thus, he must refer this procedure or speed up his technique.

BOOKING FOR PRODUCTIVITY

Time is money.
— BENJAMIN FRANKLIN

Given the example cited, it is wise to remember at all times that dentistry is a business. For this reason, we recommend not booking solidly unless each day meets the daily financial goal established for the practice. A good appointment engineer will be able to schedule non-productive procedures around productive procedures so each day reaches its established goals without creating chaos. Never allow yourself to be booked so far in advance that you are inflexible. Do not clutter the day with insignificant procedures.

It is important not to book ahead on non-productive procedures. For instance, on single-crown deliveries, we call the patient for a "seat" appointment when the crown returns from the lab. We charge the entire fee upon prepping; therefore, there is no production charged upon seating. We work these non-productive appointments into our schedule around production, enabling us still to reach our goals.

We have seen practices booked six weeks in advance. If a large case comes in, these practices cannot get it scheduled promptly. These same practices are usually low-productive practices. We have seen other practices that book four to six days ahead and do more than $100,000 per month in production. Why? They give priority to productive procedures and don't clutter the appointment book with patchwork.

Optimal scheduling means utilizing a power block protocol that schedules very productive therapy for the doctor three to four blocks each day and for the hygienist at least two blocks each day. Remember that you must have the primary dentistry to schedule.

POWER BLOCK SCHEDULING

Power blocking is the concept of scheduling primary production in one solitary time span for highest efficiency goal achievement. Up to three-quarters of the daily production goal is scheduled in the blocks. Only primary production is scheduled in this block. The book or the computer scheduler is color-coded. The power block is held open from one week to 24 hours prior to the appointment.

Block scheduling is very simple; however, it does take some effort to change from what you are doing now to this new system. Once it is working, you and your staff will find an infinite improvement over those previous patterns. The block-scheduling template allows you to start your first patient on time, have unrushed time with patients, and finish up the day on time. Being unrushed with patients and finishing up the day on time is one of the best ways to spread your reputation of care and concern for your patients.

What follows are samples of doctor and hygienist "ideal days." (Figs. 10-2 and 10-3)

The practice must decide in advance what the daily goal is and schedule accordingly. This means utilizing a *power block protocol* to fill three to four blocks with very productive therapy each day. Remember you must have the primary dentistry to schedule. When ideal scheduling protocol is routinely adhered to, the major concerns facing the system of scheduling, office running behind schedule, not finishing treatment, doing too much dentistry, and interruptions during long appointments are mostly eliminated.

	Operatory 1	Operatory 2	Operatory 3	Operatory 4
8:00	Primary			
10				
20				
30				
40				
50		Primary		
9:00				
10				
20				
30				
40	Primary			
50				
10:00				
10				
20		Primary		
30				
40				
50				
11:00				
10	Secondary			
20				
30				
40				
50				
12:00				
10				
20				
30				
40				
50				
1:00	Secondary			
10				
20				
30				
40		Insert		
50				
2:00				
10	Insert			
20				
30		Emergency		
40				
50				
3:00	New Patient			
10				
20				
30				
40				
50		Adjustment		
4:00	Consult/New Patient			
10				
20				
30				
40				
50				

Figure 10–2 Doctor's "Ideal Day" (utilizing two operatories with two assistants, one expanded functions.) Remember that scheduling effectiveness = appointment control. Scheduling effectiveness is determined by the real ratio between scheduled daily production and actual daily production.

	Operatory 1
8:00	Primary Perio
10	Root Planing Ul,Ll
20	Irrigation, OHI, Home Fl
30	Home Products
40	
50	
9:00	
10	Primary Perio
20	Root Planing Ul,Ll
30	Irrigation, OHI, Home Fl
40	Home Products
50	
10:00	
10	
20	Recare Ex, 4 BW
30	Pro, FL
40	
50	
11:00	
10	Recare Ex, 4 BW
20	Pro, FL
30	other
40	
50	
12:00	Lunch
10	
20	
30	
40	
50	
1:00	
10	Peridontal Maintain
20	Irrigation, OHI, Home Fl
30	
40	
50	
2:00	Peridontal Maintain
10	Irrigation, OHI, Home Fl
20	
30	
40	
50	
3:00	Recare
10	Exam, Fl
20	
30	
40	
50	
4:00	Recare
10	Exam, Fl
20	
30	
40	
50	

Figure 10–3 Power Block Scheduling—
Dental Hygienist "Ideal Day"

Every dental practice should determine the total chair time, not just doctor time, for each dental procedure and/or diagnostic procedure performed in the dental practice. Allow longer time with the dental hygienist at the beginning of the appointment if it is necessary to bond more with the patient or the patient has a little compliance problem. This develops high trust, and low fear. This time should be used to explain treatment to patients and make them comfortable. Be reasonable and legitimate when determining units of chair time.

Busy vs. productive—which do you prefer? It's your choice.

11 The Pulse of the Practice and Marketing

> We must make our garden grow.
> — VOLTAIRE

No practice can grow and prosper without an effective marketing program. Contrary to popular wisdom that suggests good marketing means expensive external marketing, the most successful marketing is internal marketing. It is also the most cost-effective. It begins with taking a close look at dentistry you are *not* currently offering your patients. This does not mean reinventing the wheel by going back to school to earn a new degree so that you can specialize in some esoteric area of dentistry that most patients have never heard of and don't need anyway. It does mean reviewing the basic dentistry that is the cornerstone of your practice and building on it. The easiest and least disruptive way to do this is to start with what you have and revitalize it by learning to sell benefits rather than features.

Begin by monitoring what happens in your practice. Is it a place people come to have their teeth filled, or is it a place where patients have a carefully structured recare protocol? Does the practice emphasize corrective dentistry or preventive dentistry? Do more of your patients come because something hurts or because they know that PMVs may prevent something from hurting? How many patients come for root canals and how many come for cosmetic dentistry? If your answers to these questions were fillings, corrective dentistry, pain, and root canals, your practice is selling features instead of benefits. If you want things to get better, it is time to invert the features-to-benefits ratio.

Once you decide to make the change, you must commit everyone in the practice to the decision. Just as every ship captain needs a dedicated and well-trained crew to sail a ship, every dentist needs a well-trained team to sell optimal dental care. This means that everyone in the practice must learn how to sell benefits rather than features. It means that you and the entire team must devote time and energy to letting patients know the benefits of PMVs, recare, periodontal treatment plans, and cosmetic dentistry. Your most important ally will be your dental hygienist.

Every person who comes to a dental practice is motivated by pain, fear, anxiety, financial concern, time concern, or concern about appearance. How you and your hygienist deal with these concerns is crucial. If the motivation is pain, you both need to let the patient know that preventive dentistry is the best way to prevent pain. If the motivation is financial, you both need to let the patient know that a well-designed periodontal treatment plan is a valuable investment that can preserve teeth for a lifetime and prevent expensive corrective surgery. If the motivation is anxiety or fear, you must both let the patient know that routine recare visits are always far less uncomfortable and painful than complicated corrective procedures. And while most patients will not broach the subject of appearance, human vanity is practically universal. Knowing this, you and your hygienist should promote the woefully under-utilized cosmetic benefits that can enhance every one of your patient's smiles.

The best way to market benefits rather than features is through patient education. Patients are not dental experts. You and your hygienist are, but you must both cultivate communication skills and implement scripts that fluently convey your message to patients. Neither of you can forget to include financial education in your presentations. Patients must be taught that your practice provides services that are beneficial and valuable. They must be taught that you and your hygienist are proud of your professional skills and knowledge. They must be taught that you both deserve appropriate compensation for using your skills and knowledge to keep them healthy and comfortable. Often this means walking a fine line that many dental practitioners are not comfortable with.

Overcoming this discomfort is simple if you remember one basic mantra: *explaining* fees is acceptable; *justifying* fees is unacceptable.

Learning to sell benefits instead of features can change the tone of your entire practice. It can be the strong wind that fills the sails of your ship, takes you out of the doldrums, and lets you cruise into an ocean that is alive with possibilities and potential.

Improving Productivity

A wise man will make more opportunities than he finds.
— Francis Bacon

Most patients in your practice should be coming in at least twice a year for routine checkups and routine preventive maintenance. We know this isn't always the case, but many dental professionals do not like to admit that patient non-compliance isn't always the patients' fault. Optimal dentistry has to be properly introduced and properly encouraged. The best place for this to happen is in the hygiene operatory where a four-point solution can be efficiently and comfortably instituted.

The periodontal program

All too often, your hygienist will see a patient who has not been to the office in over a year. Since 75% to 95% of all American adults have some level of periodontal disease, chances are this patient either had a previous periodontal problem, or has developed one since the last visit to your practice. With rare exceptions, the patient's gums are inflamed and the amount of harmful plaque has increased since that last visit.

Performing "just a prophy" during the new appointment is not truly serving the patient's needs. It is a stopgap solution that does not correct the underlying problem and it sends a message to the patient that skipping appointments and neglecting oral health is fine. Under these conditions, the patient is justified in thinking, "You did the same thing you did when I was coming for regular appointments, so why should I bother? I can just wait another year and come back and you'll do it again and everything will be OK."

A far better approach (for the patient and the practice) is setting up a multi-appointment periodontal therapy program. This should begin with educating the patient. "Mrs. Opossum, it has been over a year since we've seen you. Your gums are inflamed and bleeding, and there is more plaque and tartar than normal. It will take more than one appointment to take care of this."

Depending on the severity of the situation, a determination is made whether to do a full blown periodontal therapy program or just bring the patient back for one or two appointments. In either case, your hygienist will have to stress that regular office visits, coupled with proper home care, will help control the disease. Older patients must be advised of the documented relationship between periodontal disease and heart disease through handouts and other means to ensure that they understand the benefits of periodontal therapy.

Bottom line. If you have six hygiene days scheduled for every week, and just one periodontal program is instituted every other day at an average of $280 (a very conservative number and fee), this would translate into production of over $3,600 per month.

Fluoride for adults

The latest research on fluorides shows that it will kill pathogenic bacteria in plaque and reduce plaque volume. Fluoride also has an anti-inflammatory action that reduces tooth sensitivity and prevents further decay. It is just as important for adults as it is for children and can be easily instituted in the practice as part of the recare program for every patient. The long-term benefits are incalculable.

All patients can be educated on the benefits of fluoride. "Mr. Sloth, we've been receiving updated articles on the benefits of fluoride. In adults, fluoride helps kill the disease-causing bacteria, reduces tooth sensitivity, and gets down between your fillings and the teeth to prevent recurring decay. We are recommending fluoride application for patients with your situation and also for home use. Should we go ahead with the fluoride treatment today?"

Bottom line. If you have six hygiene days scheduled every week, and if two fluoride applications are done each day at an average of $19 per treatment (a conservative number of cases), this would translate into more than $1,000 per month.

Tooth whitening

Most patients' teeth grow darker with age. In our affluent society, most of us are concerned with appearance and are willing to pay for it. Many of us pay exorbitant gym fees or spend money on expensive running and walking shoes. Books on weight loss are best sellers, the cosmetic industry is booming, and hair-loss intervention products and therapies, for men and women, have flooded the market. Offering patients a beautiful smile is offering the same sort of peace of mind. Sparkling white teeth make people feel more confident and more attractive, and people who feel good about the way they look are likely to feel better emotionally and even physically.

The best way for the hygienist to approach the topic of whitening to a patient is simply to *ask*, "Ms. Vanity, have you noticed your teeth are getting darker?" She should use a shade guide to show patients where they are on the "brightness" scale and to show where whitening therapy can take them.

Patients can be given the choice of doing the whitening at home over a two–three week period or in the hygiene operatory for more instantly visible results.

Bottom line. If you have six hygiene days scheduled every week, and just one whitening case is started every other day at an average of $350 (based on a combination of home and office procedures), this would translate into production of over $4,500 per month.

Technology used to determine caries

Research has shown that many teeth with innocent occlusion "stains" are actually carious. The latest research has shown that the nature of decay has changed due to fluorides and other factors that make it harder to diagnose by looking or even by probing. With the new technology available, caries can be more easily detected and detected at the earliest stages. With microabrasion, early stage caries can be treated with no need for drilling. The appeal to patients who are frightened of needles and drills is obvious.

As with all case presentations, this one works best if it is delivered in easy to comprehend language. "The hygienist can say, "Mr. Fearful, some of your teeth have deep grooves and this is often a sign of new cavities. We have new wonderful technology to diagnose and treat cavities at the earliest stages.

Then we can remove it with our microabrasion technique in which there is no needle or drill. Let's make sure your teeth are OK."

Bottom line. If you can diagnose an average of just one carious tooth per day, this would translate to $2,500 per month!

Even with the most conservative estimates, introducing these four treatment programs and therapies can make a significant difference in the health of your patients and the health of your practice. The calculations below represent the potential for a single month:

Periodontal therapy	$3,600
Fluorides	$1,000
Whitening	$4,500
New caries	$2,500
Total	$11,600

THE OPERATORY AS A MARKETING TOOL

It takes five hundred small details to add up to one favorable impression.
— CARY GRANT

Environment matters more than you think. For this reason, your hygienist's operatory should be well stocked with marketing tools that assist patients in learning about the benefits of your practice. This includes attractive brochures on every preventive and cosmetic program and procedure that exists. The well-designed brochure about gingivitis and the beautifully illustrated brochure about porcelain veneers should be prominently displayed and should be distributed to every new patient who comes through the operatory door. The message these brochures carry should be reinforced by overhead cameras that televise before and after shots, by charts and graphs and photograph albums, and any other visual aids available. There should also be plenty of free samples that can be distributed to patients with a smile and clear, but concise instructions. These can range from flosses to toothbrushes to rinses "packaged" in a small and attractive take-home bag.

MARKETING AND THE HYGIENIST: A CASE STUDY

All patients who visit a dental practice have motivators and inhibitors that influence how they will react to the practice, the hygienist, and the treatment or procedure. These inhibitors and motivators are time, money, pain, vanity, and value. How they are addressed by the hygienist influences how likely patients will be to accept the benefits rather than merely the features offered in your practice.

A dental hygienist with a patient sitting in the operatory chair has a captive audience. A *good* dental hygienist, focusing on patient inhibitors and motivators, can get a patient to agree to all kinds of beneficial and valuable periodontal procedures and treatment programs. A *really good* dental hygienist can get a patient to agree to periodontics, cosmetics, restoration, orthodontics, and whatever else might happen to be out there.

Nothing can better illustrate just how powerful a dental hygienist's marketing potential can be than a dramatization of an ideal hygiene appointment.

Setting: The reception room of Dr. Gentletouch. Mrs. Jones, a new patient, is sitting at the edge of her seat, nervously flipping through a magazine on hiking or baking or fashion. A smiling Holly Hygienist opens the door that leads to the consulting rooms and the operatories, and walks over to Mrs. Jones, putting out a hand. Mrs. Jones half rises to take Holly's hand and gives a nervous smile as they shake hands.

Holly: Good morning, Mrs. Jones. I'm Holly and I'll be your hygienist today. I'm very happy to welcome you to our practice, and I promise I will take very good care of you. Have you filled out the little questionnaire Donna gave you?

Mrs. Jones: Yes. I have it here. *(She stands and hands the clipboard with the filled out questionnaire to Holly. She still looks anxious).*

Holly (*soothingly*): That's great. Let's go back into the examining room and we can begin. I hope we didn't keep you waiting too long.

Mrs. Jones: Oh, no. I just got the questions done and you came out here. (*Nervous laugh*) I thought I'd have at least half an hour to sit and worry and pretend to read one of the magazines out there. Isn't that how all dentists' and doctors' offices work?

Holly: (*laughing*) Not our dental office, Mrs. Jones. First of all, Dr. Gentletouch would never stand for it. But seriously, all of us here know the value of time, and we respect our patients' valuable time too much to keep them sitting in a waiting room. We're really careful to schedule appointments that we can honor.

Holly and Mrs. Jones have arrived at the door of the operatory.

Holly: Well, here we are. (*She places Mrs. Jones' questionnaire on the counter, and helps situate Mrs. Jones in the chair, covers her with a waterproof bib, etc., while chatting*). Let me just raise your chair a little here and put this bib on so we won't splash on that pretty sweater. (*She reaches for the questionnaire and sits down so that she is eye level with Mrs. Jones*). Let's look at this so I can get to know a little about your dental and medical history, okay?

Mrs. Jones: Okay.

Holly: I notice that you are not presently taking any medication. Is that correct?

Mrs. Jones: Yes.

Holly: You mention here (*points to questionnaire*) that you haven't been to see a dentist in quite some time. Is that correct?

Mrs. Jones: (*a little defensive*) Yes. Sorry, but I don't really like going to dentists and I really haven't had any problems with my teeth until last week. Well, you know how it is.

Holly: (*smiling reassuringly*). Oh, yes. We hear this from many of our patients when they first join our practice, especially if they have had a bad experience with another office in the past. I think you'll find that our practice is a little different. We really think our patient's health is important, and we do everything we can to make sure you feel comfortable with us so that you will always feel good about being here.

Holly (*turning back to clipboard*): I notice here (*she points to the questionnaire again*) that you have been experiencing a little uncomfortable puffiness in your gums and seeing a little bleeding when you brush. Is that correct?

Mrs. Jones: Yes, but only on the left side of my mouth. The right side is fine. What do you think the problem is?

Holly: Well, the best way to answer your question is to examine you. I'd like to begin by telling you what we are going to do here today. Since you haven't seen a dentist in quite some time, I suggest that we take a set of x-rays just to see if there are any problems you should know about. Is that all right with you?

Mrs. Jones: Well, I don't know. Is it going to be expensive? I mean, I have this problem with my gums and the bleeding, I don't really know if I need the x-rays.

Holly: I think it's a good idea because we can't always tell everything just from a physical examination. Sometimes puffy and bleeding gums mean there may be bone deterioration or bone loss. To give you the best treatment for this problem, we really need to see everything. We never give patients a half diagnosis because we don't think that's fair to you. If you are worried about the cost, the x-rays will be only $95 for today's visit. I believe that this entire amount or a major part of it is covered by your insurance company. We can check for you if you like.

Mrs. Jones: Yes. But isn't this going to be dangerous?

Holly: Not at all. The level of radiation is extremely low and unless a patient is pregnant or has a medical condition that specifically indicates we should not take x-rays, there is no danger whatsoever. And to make it even safer, we always use a body shield. Here let me get one for you.

Holly gets lead shield hanging on wall and places it on Mrs. Jones.

Holly: Are you comfortable with this? Can we begin taking the x-rays?

Mrs. Jones nods. Holly puts machine in position and loads the film segments into the instrument that will be inserted into the mouth. As she gets ready to take each picture, she positions film in patient's mouth and says, "now bite down a little so this stays steady." This takes a few seconds.

Holly: OK. That was the last one. Let me change the seat here, so you can sit up comfortably (*Holly adjusts chair*). Now I'm going to take these down the hall to get developed. When I come back, we can start our examination. I'll only be a minute or two and then we can start. In the meantime, I'm going to give you a couple of brochures with some information about puffiness and soreness in the gums. (*Holly pulls a couple of brochures out of a small wall rack and hands them to Mrs. Jones*). If you want to look at these while I'm gone, I'll be happy to go answer any questions when I come back. *Holly leaves room. Mrs. Jones starts looking at the brochures.*

Holly: Sorry to keep you waiting. Did you have a chance to look over the brochures? Do you have any questions?

Mrs. Jones: I guess maybe I have this gingivitis they keep talking about. I keep hearing about this on television.

Holly: Well, because of the symptoms you've told us about, this is probably true. But we will need to examine you first to see if that is really the problem and to see how much of a problem it is. What I'm going to do now is use this probe (*Holly picks one up and show it to Mrs. Jones*). See these little marks? These show us if you have pockets in the gums around your teeth. I'm going to be very gentle, but if anything I do is uncomfortable for you, please let me know. The first thing I need to do is lower your head a little so that I can see what I'm doing better. (*Holly lowers the top portion of the patient's chair*). Are you comfortable?

Mrs. Jones: Yes.

Holly: Good. Let's start over in the left side of your mouth. (*Begins working with the probe and Mrs. Jones groans immediately*). Was that too uncomfortable?

Mrs. Jones: Ouch. Is all of this going to hurt?

Holly: No. I can see that your gums in this area are extremely puffy and reddish, so we will need to hold off on the probe in this area temporarily. When Dr. Gentletouch comes in, we will talk with him about completing this part of the examination, maybe with a local anesthetic. In the meantime, let me try examining the rest of your gum tissue and we'll see what the rest of your mouth looks like. OK?

Mrs. Jones: OK. But can I stop you if it hurts?

Holly: Of course. *(Resumes probing in the other mouth areas and jots down numbers).* I'm writing down the pocket readings I'm getting here. You have a little discoloration and a little puffiness in most of the gum tissues I'm seeing, but I notice that the only area that should be really uncomfortable is that lower left section we started with. OK. That wasn't too bad was it? Let me show you what I have found.

Holly stands up and walks over to intraoral camera.

Holly: This is an intraoral camera and I'm going to let you see for yourself what I've been looking at. *(Holly shows Mrs. Jones the picture screen and the mouth lens).* This little lens takes moving pictures of your mouth and then the image is magnified and shows up on that screen up there. Let me show you how it works on that nice ring you are wearing. *(Holly points lens at ring and the image shows up on the screen)* As you can see, the camera magnifies the ring 20 to 30 times its original size. It does the same thing with your teeth and gums. This gives you and me a better opportunity to see what's going on.

Mrs. Jones: Oh, I get it.

Holly: Great. Let's get started. *(Holly inserts the camera mouthpiece in lower left quadrant first.)* Here. I'd like you to take a look at the screen. What we're looking at now is that lower left area of your mouth where you are having so much discomfort. *(Moves the camera over to the lower right quadrant).* This is more or less the same view of the lower right side of your mouth. See the difference between the two images? The gums on the right side are a little puffy and a little redder than they should be, but the gums on the left side are pretty swollen by comparison. *(Holly hands the mouthpiece to Mrs. Jones).* I'd like you to try this yourself. Move this gently from the right side back to the left again. You can pause a little in the middle so we can have a look there too.

Mrs. Jones manipulates the camera a little awkwardly at first, but then it stabilizes. She watches the images on the screen.

Holly: OK. Now if you let me have this back for a minute, I'm going to show you what else our camera does. *(She takes the mouthpiece from Mrs. Jones and moves back to the lower right quadrant).* I'm back over at the right where the gums look a little better and I'm going to fix this image and make it a picture.

Mrs. Jones: It takes pictures too?

Holly: Yes. See how the screen is divided into four sections. Well, we're going to have a different picture in each one. (*Holly clicks and the lower right quadrant is fixed on the screen*). When we're done, we'll print two sets. One for our file and one for you to take home. Now I'm going to get a picture of the lower left area that is giving you so much trouble. (*Holly clicks again*). Now let's move to the upper right. See the swelling in the gums here? Not too bad, but it needs some attention. I also notice that you have some fillings in this area. Most of them look very good. Nice work, very solid. See how well they fit the contours of your teeth? But I want you to look at something over here. (*Holly points to the far left of the screen*). See this black area? It's a very large, leaking silver filling that is probably going to fall apart completely fairly soon. You will probably need a more secure restoration here. Let me get a picture of this so we can show Dr. Gentletouch, OK? (*Holly briefly removes mouthpiece so that Mrs. Jones can reply*).

Mrs. Jones: OK. Yeah, I can really see the difference between those two and that black one. That looks pretty bad.

Holly: The filling isn't holding up too well. What would be best for the tooth would be to place a much more secure restoration, like a crown or an onlay. We'll discuss this with Dr. Gentletouch.

Mrs. Jones: Oh boy. Well, I've heard of crowns, but what's an onlay? And aren't they both expensive?

Holly: An onlay is sort of a middle step between a crown and a filling. It keeps the tooth intact. If there is enough of the original natural tooth that's intact, then we use the onlay. The onlay or crown investment is approximately $850. Most insurance companies will cover approximately 40% of this cost, but even if you have to cover a portion of this cost yourself, it's a very good investment. We are very proud of the work we do here, and the crowns and onlays we place are very strong, solid, and permanent. We've performed this procedure on many other patients and they have been delighted with the results. Mostly, it's a way to prevent more serious problems. A good restoration now can save you a lot of problems down the road. That's pretty much our philosophy here, by the way. We're committed to preventive dentistry because we know it's a better investment than corrective dentistry. Also much cheaper.

Mrs. Jones: Well, how do you know whether I need a crown or an onlay here?

Holly: Well, the x-rays will show us how much of the tooth is still intact above and below the gum line. Dr. Gentletouch will examine the tooth to confirm what we've talked about so far and to match that information precisely with the x-rays. In the meantime, let's take a picture of this tooth and then we'll continue our examination. (*Holly puts mouthpiece back in Mrs. Jones' mouth, clicks the picture, and moves mouthpiece to upper left quadrant*). Everything here looks pretty good except for the swelling. When I was working with the probe to see how deep the pockets were, this area seemed to be the healthiest. You also have a couple of fillings here, but they look good too. Let's get a picture of this too. (*Clicks again*). Now let's print these. (*Holly does so and hands one copy to Mrs. Jones*).

Mrs. Jones: Is that all then? I have this gingivitis on my left side and that bad filling on my right side.

Holly *(smiling)* : Well, that's most of it. Let me get the x-rays now and in the meantime I'd like you to take a look at these brochures. One is on crowns and one is on onlays. I've already explained the basic difference to you, but this will give you a more complete description of both procedures. When I come back, we can take a look at the x-rays and we can talk about the gingivitis and how we can handle that problem, OK?

Mrs. Jones, *taking the brochures Holly is handing her.* OK. I want to talk to you about something else too. My son Steven grinds his teeth all night long and I wanted to know if that's OK or whether he'll break them or do some other damage. His regular dentist was a pediatric guy and he just retired a few months ago, so I want to know if you take children too.

Holly: Of course. How old is your son?

Mrs. Jones: Twelve.

Holly: So he probably has all of his permanent teeth, right? Well, teeth grinding is pretty common, and you are right to be a little concerned, especially because your son is still young. We call this condition bruxism and I'm going to give you a brochure on this too. The brochure will explain the problems this condition can cause and what we can do about it. If you like, when we schedule your follow up appointments, we can schedule one for your son too. That way we can take a look a how much damage has occurred and how we can fix the damage and prevent other problems.

Mrs. Jones: Thank you. I have problems with my teeth, so I want to make sure we take good care of Steven's teeth so he won't have these problems when he's my age.

Holly: I can understand that. I have a daughter and I always want to make sure that she gets the best medical and dental care available anywhere.

Mrs. Jones: So you know how I feel.

Holly: You bet. Let me ask you something else. I see on your patient assessment form you filled in the section about smoking. I noticed when I was examining your teeth that you have a little discoloration here and there, a little yellowing. You have a really lovely smile, you know, and I wonder if you ever considered having your teeth professionally whitened?

Mrs. Jones: Well, I think about it now and then, but it's probably too expensive and if so, I have a lot of other expenses right now. I know the insurance people won't cover that one.

Holly: You're right about the insurance people, but the procedure is probably a lot less expensive than you think. There are actually two programs we offer our patients, in home or in office. Here's a little album we keep on whitening programs that were done in our office. It's just a set of before and after pictures you might want to look at. *(Holly hands Mrs. Jones the album)*. When I come back with the x-rays and the information on bruxism for you, I'll bring you some other material on our whitening programs and let you see what they involve. I'll give you a cost on both too so you can compare the information and decide which program would be best for you. Let me go get the x-rays now.

Holly leaves the room, leaving Mrs. Jones with the album on whitening and the brochures about onlays and crowns. Mrs. Jones places the brochures in her lap and looks at the album. Then Holly returns to the operatory with the x-rays, the brochure on bruxism, and an office fact sheet on whitening.

Holly: Well, here we are. I see you've been checking out our little before and after album. What do you think?

Mrs. Jones: What a difference! I saw before teeth there that looked a lot worse than mine and the change was really something. Are these pictures real?

Holly: Oh yes. These are actual patients who had the treatments under our care. We have letters from some of them after the treatment—I have copies of a couple of them here and the other information I promised to get you. I'm glad you are interested and I think you'll be delighted with the results. We're very proud of our whitening program, you know, because we always want our patients to feel their best and look their best too. When Dr. Gentletouch comes to examine you, I'll let him know that you are interested in a whitening treatment and he'll be happy to talk with you about this too.

Mrs. Jones: OK.

Dr. Gentletouch enters the room. Holly places the first x-ray on backlighted screen and points.

Dr. Gentletouch: First I want to show you that tooth that Holly was concerned about, the one that Holly says needs a better and more secure restoration. *(Doctor hands Mrs. Jones the photo taken with the intraoral camera).* On this photo you can see what it looks on the outside. If you look at the x-ray image you can see what it looks like on the inside. *(Points with a pencil to the specific x-ray area).* The x-ray shows that filling is in pretty bad shape, but we also have some good news. The tooth has not cracked and there is actually quite a large tooth area that is still intact. This means that we will be able to insert an onlay and that a crown will not be necessary. The x-ray also shows that the problem has not yet begun to impact the root area, so if the procedure is done soon, we won't have to worry about a root canal.

Mrs. Jones: Well, that really is good news. I've been sitting here worrying that you would tell me I needed a root canal and a crown and all I could see was pain and dollar signs. So if I have this onlay, it will stop the problem and it will only cost me about $850?

Holly: That's right. And, as I mentioned before, your insurance may cover some of that cost and it may not. But I also want to emphasize that this procedure should be done quickly so that the condition doesn't deteriorate.

Mrs. Jones: Oh, I agree.

Holly: Good. Then we'll have the receptionist discuss financial arrangements and schedule an appointment for you to have this done as soon as possible.

Dr Gentletouch: Now, let's discuss the other dental concern that Holly found today. (*Puts all x-rays on backlighted screen in the shape of mouth clockwise: (left upper quadrant, right upper quadrant, right lower quadrant and left lower quadrant).*

Mrs. Jones: Uh-oh. This is where you're going to tell me about this gingivitis and how my whole mouth is falling apart and I'm going to have to get dentures, right?

Dr. Gentletouch: Well, I'm not going to suggest anything that terrible, but I am going to talk to you seriously about the gum problems that you have and tell you what we should do about them. First, let's look at these pictures. (*Points to lower left quadrant*). This is the area that I'm most concerned about because it shows extensive periodontal disease – that's gum disease. What has happened here is that the gum area has become infected and has created a problem with the teeth in this area and the underlying bone structure too. Your gums are causing you a lot of surface discomfort, but what's going on under the gum line is even more of a concern because it really can cause you to lose all your teeth in this area. If you look at the other three x-rays, you see that the bone structure in those other three looks a lot more solid. This is a very good sign because it shows that the major deterioration has occurred only in this lower left area. But if you look at the pictures we took with intraoral camera, you'll see that the gums in these three areas are also showing signs of irritation and swelling.

Mrs. Jones: Oh great. Now what? Can you fix this or should I just have all my teeth pulled and get dentures?

Dr. Gentletouch: Well, first I would like to tell you that our priority here is to make sure our patients keep their own teeth for a lifetime, if it is at all possible. From what I am seeing here, all of these teeth can be saved, even the ones in this lower left quadrant, if we take some very strong and very quick action here.

Mrs. Jones: So what do you do?

Dr. Gentletouch: Holly will discuss your periodontal therapy. I will leave you in her good hands, and look forward to seeing you very soon.

Holly: The first thing we do is place you in a periodontal treatment program. We'll begin with that left lower area where the most damage has occurred and the process we use here is called root planing. This means we go deep down into the root area of each tooth and clean any plaque and take care of any infection that is below the gum line. This procedure is done under local anesthesia if you wish, so there is little or no discomfort afterwards. When we clean up this area, the tissues have a chance to heal. In many cases, they begin to grow back around the root areas and this stops the teeth from wobbling and also stops the progressive deterioration of the bones underneath. The bone loss that has already happened cannot be reversed, but we can make sure that it doesn't get worse.

Mrs. Jones: What about the other sections of my mouth. Do you have to do this root planing there too?

Holly: No, from what I see, there is some periodontal disease in these areas, but it has not progressed as badly as in that lower left area that is giving you so much trouble. The treatment here is some scaling to take care of the plaque. We recommend strongly that all patients with any level of gum disease come in for preventive maintenance appointments three or four times a year once they commit to the periodontal therapy. This way we can keep the disease under control. We will also give you home care instruction so that you can be a partner in this. What you do at home between visits is going to be a very important part of the treatment program.

Mrs. Jones: Like what?

Holly: Well, to begin with, what you do at home is going to make a big difference in what happens when you come to the office. So we are going to give you some pointers on brushing and flossing to keep your teeth and gums in better condition. We will also suggest a therapeutic mouth rinse, an electric toothbrush, and an irrigation system that will clean below the gum line.

Mrs. Jones: You know, I looked at this brochure while you were gone and it says some scary things about this infection. This Surgeon General thing, for example ...can I really get a heart attack or cancer if we don't do this?

Holly *(soothingly):* Well, we didn't want to scare you, but one of the things that has come to the attention of the medical community recently is that many things that happen in the mouth *can and do* affect the rest of the body. Periodontal disease, unfortunately, is one of the biggest areas of concern because the bacteria, which come from infected gums can be easily spread to other organs and tissues through the bloodstream. With really severe infections, this bacteria can cause a lot of damage. Because we really care about our patients being healthy and safe, we feel we should be honest with them about this, even if it is a little scary. That's one of the reasons why we are so committed to preventive dentistry, including a really solid maintenance program. If we can stop diseases from getting worse or prevent problems before they occur, we are doing the best thing we can to keep our patients in good health.

Mrs. Jones: Boy, it looks like I should have come to see you a lot sooner. I didn't realize my mouth was in such bad shape.

Holly: Mrs. Jones, no one in our office believes in making people feel bad about their past dental history. We are just glad that you came to us now, because every problem that we discussed today has a solution and we are glad that we will be working with you to make things better. You aren't the first patient to come into our office with these problems, and believe me, some of the dental and periodontal problems we've seen in first time patients has been much worse than what I've seen today. Much worse. But all of the patients that have stayed with the treatment programs we set up are much happier and much healthier than when they first came to see us. I know that this will happen with you, too. Let's review your proposed treatment plan, now, shall we?

In just one visit, our expert hygienist has succeeded in establishing a need, instilling a value, and asking for a commitment. She has educated the patient about oral health and about financial arrangements. She has managed to promote a treatment plan for the patient's periodontal condition, has recommended a whitening procedure, and has recruited a new patient, the patient's son Steven, to the practice. We can safely assume that Mr. Jones will start visiting the practice before too long, along with assorted friends and colleagues and neighbors. No amount of money invested in external marketing can begin to measure up to what has occurred in this scenario.

12 New Horizons

> *The riders in a race do not stop*
> *short when they reach the goal.*
> *There is a little finishing canter.*
> — OLIVER WENDELL HOLMES

The first 11 chapters of this book presented guidelines for creating and developing an excellent hygiene department that functions as a semi-autonomous unit in a master dental practice. In each of these chapters, evidence has been presented, case studies have been cited, and suggestions have been made for design and implementation of the new hygiene paradigm. Scripts and forms have been provided for illustrative purposes; in rare instances, cautionary notes have been appended for emphasis.

All books reach an end point, a conclusion, which in its lowest form is a summation of that which came before and in its highest form serves as a prediction of what is yet to come. Occasionally, the two forms cannot be separated because that which was, is an inherent part of that which is to be. This is the case in concluding *Dental Hygiene: The Pulse of the Practice.*

The Introduction to this book begins with a broad definition of dental hygiene as "the field of dentistry that is based on preserving and maintaining oral health. Concerned with keeping the teeth and gums in healthy condition, dental hygiene is more and more defined in terms of preventive care that provides protection against oral diseases as well as other diseases that affect the human body." The entire book revolves around this definition—every chapter in the book supports or relies upon this basic premise. And so, despite detours and deviations, the wheel has come full circle.

As we have all heard, understanding where we have been helps us know where we are and where we are going. This applies to dental hygiene as well as history. To see the future of dental hygiene, therefore, we must revisit the past and revisit, as well, the insights of the individuals who brought dental hygiene from the shadows into the limelight.

From the Greek and Arabian physicians of antiquity, from Alfred C. Fones who trained the first "official" hygienists in his garage, from the American Dental Hygiene Association which was founded in 1923, and from Surgeon General David Satcher, we have learned that prevention is the secret ingredient of oral health and total health. We have learned, as well, that cooperation and coordination are often the most important components of success in any endeavor. It is in combining these two truths that we have created the focus of this concluding chapter.

PREVENTIVE PARTNERSHIP: THE ROAD TO EXCELLENCE

Revolutions do not go backward.
— ABRAHAM LINCOLN

We have already posited that making the hygiene department the pivotal force of a dental practice is a revolutionary concept. But in order to make the revolution succeed, the hygiene department must move forward. This forward momentum can be sustained only as a cooperative venture that is aided, abetted, and supported by multiple advocates. It is the hygienist who must take primary responsibility in building the coalition that can make this happen.

The first members of this powerful coalition, naturally, should be the dental team in every individual practice. In chapter 5, we explained in detail how everyone from the dentist to the dental assistant to the receptionist to the billing clerk has a supporting role in assisting the hygienist in presenting to patients a case for optimal preventive dentistry. But no dental practice exists in a vacuum, and by logical extension, the hygienist and the dental practitioner need to form strong alliances within the dental community as a whole to further this aim. This means establishing and nurturing strong working ties with professional organizations that have the numbers and the authority to arm the revolutionaries with legitimacy, thus strengthening the revolution itself and the dental profession as a whole. Organizations like the American Dental Association, the American Academy of Periodontology, the American Dental Hygiene Association, the American Academy of General Dentistry, and the American Association of Dental Assistants can be strong allies and can assist oral hygiene in its quest to form further alliances in this great cause.

Next on board should be members of the medical profession at large. Every physician representing every medical specialty should by this time be at least marginally aware of the mouth-body connection described so meticulously in the report of the Surgeon General. Yet dentistry continues to be viewed by many as the lesser twin or the younger sibling of the medical profession. It is up to every hygienist to dispel this misconception by making certain that every cardiologist, every pediatrician, every obstetrician, and every other medical specialist or generalist is fully apprised of how those respective specialties are impacted by oral health and how great an ally they have in hygiene.

Especially not to be neglected in forming these alliances are practitioners specializing in nutrition and geriatrics. With much of the nation already attuned to the healthful nature of certain foods and the detrimental nature of others with respect to cholesterol, obesity, anti-carcinogens, and fats, hygienists have a forum that can easily accommodate information about nutritional choices that bolster good oral health. As America's baby boomers age, hygienists will be called upon to help deal with the growing issue of age-related oral health problems in a variety of ways. The message of prevention carries weight even when oral health habits of a lifetime have spawned severe problems.

While seeking to create partnerships with established traditional dental and medical individuals, organizations and institutions, it is wise to remember that there is much to be learned from other revolutionaries. While custom and security often dictate that what is well known is best, it is worth investigating the lesser known. Every hygienist should invest some time in researching whether alternatives such as acupuncture, homeopathic medication and anti-microbial therapy, whole body dentistry, or the use of chemo-therapeutic agents, promulgated by those not yet fully endorsed by the dental, medical, and scientific community at large, have something to offer.

Professional cooperation between medicine, dentistry, and the United States Surgeon General's Office can and will lead to additional partnerships, the most important of which is the partnership with patients. Several chapters of this book are devoted in whole or in part to patient education. While a hygienist with excellent communication skills is the foot soldier best suited to building a case for good oral health and preventive dentistry, she should not have to do so alone. She should have behind her legions and battalions led by courageous commanders who are willing to fight the good fight with her, willing to support her, and willing to promote the ideas she imparts to patients. Some patients already listen to what their hygienists have to say. How many more might listen (and listen better) if the hygienist's ideas were ideas universally promoted in every sphere of dentistry and medicine is incalculable.

While seeking the support of the entire dental and medical profession to help create a partnership with patients, the hygienist can never forget her own strength and her own potential in forging ties with patients. Nothing can match chair side case presentation. But the hygienist's presentations should not be limited to the operatory. Community outreach in myriad directions should be a given. A few examples should suffice.

Every hygienist who speaks with patients about the connection between oral health and total health is equally capable of disseminating this information outside the box and outside of the operatory. Every school in the nation, every chamber of commerce, and countless professional and self-help organizations invite guest speakers to present on a variety of topics for a variety of reasons. Most create and maintain a "potential speakers list" which is consulted and put to a vote by a committee. The decision to choose one speaker or another is always subjective, but in many cases the speaker has satisfied one of the following criteria: fame, timely information, novelty, useful information about health concerns, or useful information about money. Any hygienist reviewing this list of criteria should respond with, "I may not be famous, but I sure can talk about all that other stuff." The next action is for her to make a phone call and volunteer her services as a guest speaker. The possibilities are endless, and a speaker at one event is quite likely to be asked to speak at another.

Reaching out to the community can lead to many other alliances. Municipal outreach programs may welcome innovative and helpful hygienists who volunteer their time and energy to teaching and promoting oral health in a variety of venues. In some instances, mobile dentistry units have created a wonderful opportunity for hygienists to contribute their professional skills while spreading the word about the power of prevention.

In this country, mass media is a powerful tool for disseminating information and for shaping public opinion. Forming a partnership with a newspaper or radio or television reporter can further improve your power to educate people about preventive dentistry. If, for example, your hygienist has been invited to present a seminar at a PTA meeting or at a luncheon for local small business owners concerned about the cost of dental insurance, make it news by making it known to the news media. Quite recently, evening news programs have begun inserting medical alerts, information about medical research, or timely medical hints and tips. The media does not create these sound bites from whole cloth— the information is provided by physicians and dentists and others who are considered trusted sources. A phone call or a well-scripted letter to an editor or a news anchor may lead to interesting opportunities.

The insurance industry may seem an unlikely bedfellow in this coalition for prevention, yet even here a resourceful hygienist can make a difference. Many insurers are reluctant to cover preventive maintenance costs or periodontal procedures that they deem out of the range of "usual and ordinary." While the idea of combating the vested interests of insurance companies by actively pushing for a redefinition of "usual and ordinary" may seem akin to performing the labors of Hercules, it is a task that no hygienist should ignore. Consider the times you have heard a patient say, "I'll get the dentistry if the insurance covers it." How difficult it is to fight this comment and others like it! But the difficulty can be ameliorated if a hygienist recognizes that convincing the patient that prevention is better than correction is only half the battle. The other half is convincing insurers that their short-sighted "usual and ordinary" may actually be costing them in the long run. All too often, those same patients who do not have preventive oral treatments because of their insurance carriers' regulations will return to a practice for extensive and expensive corrective emergency procedures that the insurance carriers must pay for.

In dealing with these issues, a hygienist working alone may accomplish very little. Hygienists working as a unit with the strength of the ADHA, the AGP, the ADA, and the AAP behind them can accomplish much more. Hygienists enlisting the aid of their patients can do wonders. Every hygienist can work with patients to inform them about the difference between prophylactic and corrective procedures. Every hygienist can ask patients to actively lobby insurance companies who do not cover prophylactic procedures to change their range of coverage. Every American understands the power of a strong and vocal lobby in improving and protecting the rights of consumers. Your patients are no exception, and if recruited, can be tremendously influential in this matter.

In a related matter, a poll taken by the American Dental Association in 2000 revealed that lack of insurance coverage was the top reason for not visiting dentists, a fact that should present to hygiene a new opportunity for creating a partnership with the business community. Most employers provide their employees with health insurance. Most employers do *not* provide a dental plan in this package, citing excessive cost. And yet the cost of not providing dental coverage and thus discouraging preventive dentistry is exceedingly high. Independent studies conducted by the Coalition for Oral Health and the American Fund for Dental Health Association (see the ADHA report on *The Future of Oral Health*, 2001) reported that Americans lost between 20 and 30 million work days or school days annually because of oral health problems. By how many millions of days could these figures be reduced if business and industry recognized that preventive oral health care, covered by dental insurance, is more cost effective for everyone concerned? How many millions of dollars the business community could save by becoming active partners in prevention is a statistical projection well worth investigating.

School days missed because of oral health problems suggest that we review a piece of ancient history in American dentistry, specifically, the 1870 meeting of the American Dental Association, at which it was decided that school textbook publishers devote space to proper oral health care. And we should likewise recall that the first graduates of Alfred C. Fones' hygiene classes went into public schools to ensure that children were taught good oral care health habits. Perhaps it is time to renew and strengthen our partnership with

America's schools. Today, every school system in the country incorporates health education into its curriculum. The question arises as to what percentage of health education is devoted to oral health. An even greater question is whether anyone out there is teaching the children of America that oral health and general health are related. Who is better suited than the dental hygienist in creating educational material that will fill the void? It can be presented at school assemblies, at PTA meetings, at teacher in-service days, at pedagogical conferences and conventions, and at numerous other high impact venues. Reaching children may be the most important reaching a dental hygienist does, for it is in childhood that habits are acquired and it is in childhood that good oral health habits should be grounded. Children who learn the right and proper way to care for their teeth and gums at an early age will become adults with healthy teeth and gums. Here indeed is a partnership for life!

In a discussion of partnerships for prevention, we cannot forget the tremendous potential of technology. We have already discussed in some detail the obvious benefits of the intraoral camera, but it is worth mentioning the positive impact of other technology as well. Digital radiography, for example, is fast replacing traditional x-ray equipment because it is easier, quicker, and more versatile. Electric toothbrushes and home irrigation systems, once novelties, are now standard home-care equipment for millions. Computer technology has changed the world and the changes have spilled over into dental practices. A dental hygienist, once armed with only a scaler, can now be armed with a sophisticated operatory computer that can assist her in diagnosis, record maintenance, and countless other ways. A computer can also be used as an ideal way of communicating with patients in their homes. Patients' questions can be answered electronically, either by email or through websites developed and maintained by the hygienist as a means of promoting preventive dentistry. Do not underestimate the appeal a user-friendly hygiene website can have for young patients weaned on computer technology, especially if the site is interactive and even more so if your young patients are recruited as contributors.

A partnership with computer technology presents a host of other benefits, including an opportunity to research new and creative developments in the profession. It may also be an inducement for the hygienist to participate more actively in conducting research activities of her own.

The ADHA, founded in 1923 to provide resources, information, and a group identity for dental hygienists, continues to perform these functions. But it has evolved into an organization that provides its members with many other benefits, including a platform from which to launch independent scientific research related to dental hygiene. The ADHA Code of Ethics, in fact, lists in its Standards of Professional Responsibility a specific paradigm for scientific investigation. It instructs hygienists "to conduct research that contributes knowledge that is valid and useful to our clients."

With the backing of the ADHA and the infinite resources made available through computer technology, every hygienist has the opportunity to become involved in research. The research activities need not take her far from home or far from the practice. Hygienists, for example, know what works chair side and what doesn't. They know what would make things run more smoothly, more comfortably, more efficiently, and more productively. Each of them has the potential to create solutions or investigate better working alternatives. Each has the potential to invent and patent that better mousetrap.

The unprecedented scientific, medical, dental, and technological advances of the previous century provide merely a glimmer of what human beings are capable of conceiving and creating. We cannot predict what the future holds, but we can help shape that future by being always willing to learn and explore the world around us. In dental hygiene, as in life, the passive and complacent will reap mediocrity. It is for those who dare that the future holds infinite promise.

Index

A

B

Bad blood theory, xiv

Baltimore College of Dental Surgery, xv-xvi

Benefits package, 29

Booking for productivity, 182-183

Broken appointments, 17, 159-164

Buffer conflict, 48

C

Camera (intraoral), 103-106

Cancellations, 17, 163-164

Care objectives (doctor), 118-120

Care objectives (hygienist), 121-124: communication form, 123

Career information, xvi-xix, 1-2

Caries incidence, 78

Caries technology, 191-192

Case acceptance, 17, 85-87, 106-107

Case presentation, 101-102

Case study (hygienist marketing), 193-205

Caustic dentifrice, xiv

Chart auditing (recare), 155-159: reactivation call, 158; exit interview, 158-159; unhappy patient, 159

Children (5-9), 78

China, xiv

Classified ads (hygienist), 25

Closure statements, 86-87

Code of Ethics, 24-25, 49, 77-78

Commission compensation, 30-31

Commitment, 7-8

Communication, 38, 47, 74, 93-114, 123, 140-141: pearls, 74, 108-114

Compliance (patient), 136-141: failure factors, 137-140; denial, 137-138; fear, 138-139; money, 139; patient dissatisfaction, 139-140; improving compliance, 140-141; record, 141

Compliance improvement, 140-141: communication, 140-141

Compliance record, 141

Comprehensive exam, 89-91

Constructive criticism, 48

Content (annual retreats), 71-73: annual review, 72; agenda, 72-73

Continuing education, 29

Controlled periodontitis, 131

Creativity, 47

Crisis management, 55

Criticism, 48

Culture (office), 46

Customer service, 18

D

Decision support, 47

Defeat (learning from), 57

Denial factor, 137-138

Dental assistant, 44

Dental hygiene department/program, xi, xiii-xix, 1-9, 89-114: profit and productivity, 2-4; vision, 4-5; setting goals, 5-6; achieving goals, 6-7; purpose development, 7-8; philosophy of practice, 8-9; mission statement, 8-9; empowerment, 89-114

Dental hygienist, 45, 52-54, 85-87: performance appraisal, 52-54

E

F

G

Preventive maintenance visit, 17, 92-93

Production efficiency (scheduling), 174-175

Productivity goals, 179-181

Productivity improvement, 189-192: periodontal program, 189-190; fluoride for adults, 190; tooth whitening, 191; technology (caries), 191-192

Productivity, 2-4, 68, 174-175, 179-183, 189-192: scheduling, 174-175; goals, 179-181; improvement, 189-192

Professional fulfillment, 50-55: growth appraisal, 51; employee performance appraisal, 52-54; practice growth and success, 55

Professional partnership, xi, 1-2, 208-214

Profit/profitability, 2-4, 68-69

Punctuality, 35

Purpose (annual retreat), 71-73: annual review, 72; agenda, 72-73

Purpose (meeting), 61

Purpose development (practice), 7-8

R

Radiographic policy, 136

Ratings for job duties, 54

Reactivation (recare), 153-159: sample letters, 153-154; chart auditing, 155-159; calling, 158

Recare appointment increase, 151-154

Recare, retention, and hygiene, 18, 147-171: department assessment, 148; hygiene recare efficiency, 149; pearls, 150; pre-appointment recare system, 150-151; appointment increase, 151-154; reactivation letters, 153-154; chart auditing, 155-159; broken appoint-

ments, 159-164; cancellations, 163-164; patient loss, 165-171

Refractory periodontitis, 125

Restorative dentistry, xi

Retention (patient), 18, 147-171: patient loss, 165-171

Retreats, 70-73: date/place/time, 71; purpose/content, 71-73

Rewards (performance), 52

S

Safety, 33-34

Salary, 28-29: continuing education, 29; benefits package, 29

Schedule review, 69

Scheduling, 69, 173-186: schedule review, 69; objectives, 173-174; production efficiency, 174-175; time management, 176-178, 181-182; patient call list, 178; hygienist scheduling, 179; productivity goals, 179-181; time allowance per procedure, 181-182; booking for productivity, 182-183; power blocking, 183-186; ideal day, 184

Scripts, 85-87: philosophy, 85; permission, 86; need and motivation, 86; closure statements, 86-87

Sealant use, 78

Self-appreciation, 56

Self-assessment (patient), 83-84

Staff meeting, 64

Strategies, 1-9

Success sharing, 57

Sumeria, xiii

T

Team meeting, 63

Teamwork/team spirit, 35, 37-57: team player, 35, 54-55; communication, 38; positive vs. negative, 38; office procedures/protocol, 38-39; office manual pearls, 40-45; management pearls, 46-49; professional fulfillment, 50-55; attitude pearls, 56-57

Technology (caries), 191-192

Time allowance per procedure, 181-182

Time management, 35, 176-178, 181-182: time allowance per procedure, 181-182

Tissue control, 116

Tooth decay, xiii-xvii

Tooth whitening, 191

Tooth worm theory, xiii-xiv

Tooth/gum disease (history), xiii-xvii

Transitions, 11-20: practice evaluation, 12-16; vital signs, 12-13; visualization, 17-18; motivation, 18-20

Treatment explanation pearls, 93

Treatment plan (periodontal), 128

Trend (preventive dentistry), 207-214

Trust your judgment, 57

U

U.S. Surgeon General's report, xviii-xix, 17, 76-77

Unhappy patient, 159

United States, xv-xix: history, xv-xvi

V

Vision (professional), 4-5

Visualization of practice, 17-18

Vital signs, 12-13: dentist, 12; dental hygienist, 12-13

W

Whitening, 191

Working interview, 22-23

Y

Young adults (19-39), 80